Winner of the 2007 Natalie Davis Spingarn Writer's Award
— National Coalition for Cancer Survivorship

"*Nordie's at Noon* is an honest and inspiring testament to
[these authors'] experiences which, I am completely confident . . .
will inspire thousands of women as it inspired me."
—Elizabeth Edwards

"[A] funny, poignant, and exceedingly valuable resource."
— *Library Journal*

". . . This is a rare book that has the saddest of endings and yet still
manages to be—yes—life affirming." —*People* (4 stars)

"A warm and intimate detailing of how cancer upends young lives."
—Ms. *Magazine*

"Whether you're a woman who has herself been affected by
breast cancer or a man who is as healthy as a horse, *Nordie's at Noon*
is a lesson in the importance of treasuring friends and family,
finding your inner strength, and embracing each day as a gift,
if only because there may not necessarily be a tomorrow."
—*Philadelphia Inquirer*

"An emotional, touching and even funny memoir about how
these women bonded over facing breast cancer together."
—LifetimeTV.com

"*Nordie's at Noon* provides something for everyone dealing with
breast cancer — and further explores what so many of us already
know—that true friendship can see us through just about anything!"
—TheBreastCareSite.com

"A celebration of friendship and living life to the fullest."
—*Today's Chicago Woman*

"*Nordie's at Noon* is a wonderful read with a weighty message:
all women need to be actively concerned about their breast health,
not just in October, but all year long."
— *Health News Digest*

"The story of how these amazing women faced and fought cancer at a young age is as real as it gets. They spare no details, make us cry and laugh, and most important, they give great hope to any woman facing the disease, as well as to the husband or boyfriend who stands by her side." —Marc Silver, author of *Breast Cancer Husband*

"*Nordie's at Noon* is a warm and moving testament to friendship and to the bonds forged in the authors' battle against breast cancer. I highly recommend it for women of all ages, particularly college women and their parents who need to understand that breast cancer can happen to them." —Becky H. Kirwan, President, Zeta Tau Alpha Foundation, Inc.

"The authors of *Nordie's at Noon* were able to capture the gamut of emotions young women face while battling breast cancer in their poignant writing. By having the courage to write about their experiences, they have given those who care for young women diagnosed with breast cancer an opportunity to better serve this unique patient population." — Sheryle A. D'Amico, MHA, Director, Oncology Center and Breast Center at Lawrence Memorial Hospital

"*Nordie's at Noon* is a must read for everybody. The experiences and insights of these four incredible women will bring about a fresh new perspective for each reader." —Karin McCrary, RN, Former Director of the Breast Center at Menorah Medical Center

"The(se) four courageous women...have given us a rare, personal, and very intimate picture of what it is like to experience a devastating diagnosis at such a young age. Their...journey serves to inform and empower the reader to take the unwanted diagnosis of cancer as an opportunity to not only survive, but to thrive. Even with this unwelcome intruder of cancer in their lives and the uncertainty of possible death as the outcome, their spirit, their wisdom, and their courage prevail throughout the pages of this inspiring book." —Ellen Stovall, President and CEO, National Coalition for Cancer Survivorship

Make today count!!

Kim
Beckley

NORDIE'S
at Noon

The Personal Stories of Four Women
"Too Young" for Breast Cancer

Patti Balwanz
Kim Carlos
Jennifer Johnson
Jana Peters

Da Capo
∞
LIFE
LONG

A Member of the Perseus Books Group

Copyright © 2006 by NaNoon, LLC

Designed by Trish Wilkinson
Set in 11.5-point Goudy by the Perseus Books Group

Library of Congress Cataloging-in-Publication Data

Nordie's at noon : the personal stories of four women too young for breast cancer / Patti Balwanz . . . [et al.]. — 1st Da Capo Press ed.
   p. cm.
   HC: ISBN-10: 0-7382-1086-2; ISBN-13: 978-0-7382-1086-5
   PBK: ISBN-10: 0-7382-1112-5; ISBN-13: 978-0-7382-1112-1 1. Breast—
Cancer—Patients—Biography. 2. Breast—Cancer—Anecdotes. I. Balwanz, Patti, d. 2003.
RC280.B8N67 2006
362.196'9944900922—dc22   2006021043

First Da Capo Press edition 2006
First Da Capo Press paperback edition 2007

Published by Da Capo Press
A member of the Perseus Books Group
www.dacapopress.com

Da Capo Press books are available at special discounts for bulk purchases in the U.S. by corporations, institutions, and other organizations. For more information, please contact the Special Markets Department at the Perseus Books Group, 2300 Chestnut Street, Suite 200, Philadelphia, PA 19103, or call (800) 255-1514, or e-mail special.markets@perseusbooks.com

10 9 8 7 6 5 4 3 2 1

Nordie's at Noon is dedicated to
Patti Balwanz and Jana Peters—our friends,
sisters, co-authors, and inspirations.

Jen and Kim

Contents

Foreword

This year in the United States, more than 214,000 women will be diagnosed with breast cancer. The American Cancer Society estimates that 1 of every 7 women in the United States will be affected by breast cancer in their lifetimes. Although the median age for breast cancer is sixty-three, breast cancer will affect 1 out of every 229 women in their thirties and 1 of every 3,000 pregnancies.

Despite these overwhelming statistics, there is a paucity of information available for women younger than thirty-five with breast cancer. The issues that affect women at various stages in their lives are different. In our twenties and thirties, we deal with issues of career development, dating, marriage, children. In our forties and fifties, we deal with balancing choices, change, and the maintenance of our homes, careers, and ourselves. And in our sixties and seventies, we move on to nurturing and relishing the choices we have made in our lives. Superimposing a diagnosis of breast cancer into each of these various stages carries a vast array of challenges.

The "Nordie Girls" (Patti, Jana, Jennifer, and Kim) have written a remarkable book. Each has captured a different perspective of the challenges of having breast cancer when younger than thirty-five. Individually, each of these women is extraordinary. Collectively through their friendship and their shared experience, they have created a beautifully written book.

As a breast surgeon, I have had the privilege of participating in the direct care of more than twelve hundred breast cancer patients. Among them, these four young women stand out. Anyone who has met Patti, Jana, Jen, or Kim knows what I mean. They are unforgettable.

Being a physician to each of these amazing young women has been pure joy and a difficult challenge. Trying to slow them down long enough for appropriate healing and recovery felt like holding down four balloons in a hurricane. These "Gen X" young women are all multitasking overachievers . . . each competing with herself to better her own best. Thanks to their cell phones, iPods, and Internet communications, these women came to their appointments fully armed with the latest information. Our discussions were always fascinating and rich. Usually, they would turn the conversation to their concerns about each other rather than about themselves.

When I first met Patti seven years ago, she struck me as an extremely poised woman for her age. At that time, she was twenty-four years old and striking in her manner. Despite her high-powered business attire, she exuded fun and bubbled with joy. It seemed to be a rare combination. When Patti entered the room, she didn't merely "walk" in her high-heeled pumps . . . she "bounced."

It is my practice to meet in person with the patient and her husband or family when a pathology report reveals a malignancy. Patti arrived for this discussion of treatment options with two of her good friends! At first, this struck me as odd. Certainly, I thought, this young woman *must* have a parent or family member who is interested in her care. I was concerned that Patti did not have a supportive family. Several days later, after meeting her loving and devoted parents, I realized that this was the first of many "Patti-isms." I soon learned to accept and cherish these "Patti-isms." Patti had a truly independent "I can handle anything . . . bring it on!" attitude. Her ability to bounce through life earned her the nickname Tigger.

Jana was twenty-seven years old when she was diagnosed with breast cancer. She was engaged to be married and work- ing in a challenging and exciting job. Life was good. Jana en- joys life . . . enjoys having fun . . . riding roller coasters . . . having pedicures . . . shopping for those perfect pink acces- sories. She can be intense and professional in her research work and very organized while running a foundation board meeting—and then, one minute later, she can be full of gig- gles! Jana has an infectious laugh—the kind that doesn't allow you to take yourself too seriously. I cannot remember a single encounter with Jana when I haven't laughed. Despite my protests, throughout her treatment, Jana kept a whirlwind pace. Her job involved frequent travel around the country. I learned never to assume she was in Kansas City. Her nick- name, Jana Banana, seemed to fit her. Healthy, tropical, fruity! In addition, Jana is the kind of person who dreams with the innocence of a child and then, with goal-setting and drive, she makes those dreams a reality.

At age twenty-seven, Jennifer was living the ideal life. Mar- ried to a wonderful man, involved in a rewarding career, start- ing her family. In many ways, Jennifer was "the girl next door." Sweet, smiling, friendly. The kind of person whom everyone cherishes as a best friend. Always giving, always thoughtful, organized, and punctual. A person you could count on. I had heard about Jen long before I met her. Many mutual acquaintances had asked me about their young friend . . . a woman who had been diagnosed with breast cancer while pregnant. Several years after her diagnosis, she became my patient.

When I learned of her friendship with Patti and Jana, I felt they would complement one another beautifully. Secretly, I was thrilled to find a trustworthy ally to help me try to keep bouncing Tigger and jet-setting Jana grounded!

Kim was married to her high school sweetheart and was the mother of a young son. She was thirty when she was diagnosed with breast cancer. Poised, striking, articulate . . . the kind of person who looks you in the eye when she speaks. Kim had done all her homework, and always arrived for her consultation with facts in hand. She knew all the statistics. With true grit and determination, she came with a pure "I am *not* going to let this cancer beat me . . . no way . . . no how" attitude. Kim is an amazing woman. From the start, she was on a mission to get the word out to inform others and to make the road easier for other breast cancer patients. Kim doesn't think of the world with boundaries. When trying to make a difference, she doesn't think locally . . . or regionally. She thinks globally! Together with Patti, Jana, and Jen, Kim made the circle complete.

It has been a privilege and honor to know Patti, Jana, Jen, and Kim through their medical care and through their friendship. Yet I learned more about their experience with cancer in reading this book than I ever knew through participating in their health care. I would highly recommend this book to all young women faced with a diagnosis of breast cancer and to their support teams, their significant others, their friends, and their families. I would also recommend this book to persons on the health care team caring for young women with breast cancer, including primary physicians, gynecologists, surgeons, oncologists, radiation oncologists, nurses, and others. This book provides a brilliant insight into the collective thoughts and feelings of young women battling this disease.

Sharing in the journeys of my breast cancer patients has taught me many priceless lessons. Among these, two lessons stand out. I have learned that a diagnosis of breast cancer will not define you. How you handle the diagnosis will define your character. Also, breast cancer is not meant to change your life. It will merely amplify the life you already have. Through this book, you will see four beautiful examples of these lessons—lessons learned and lessons lived.

When faced with a challenge, some people respond by withdrawing; others maintain; and yet others find the spirit to rise above themselves—not only to persevere but to triumph. This book is a beautiful testimony to that spirit and to the extraordinary women who shared the stories recounted in *Nordie's at Noon*.

Amie Jew, M.D.
Breast Surgeon

Preface:
Bosom Buddies

It all began at "Nordie's," the trendy café in the Nord-strom department store. There, the four of us would meet for lunch the last Tuesday of each month. The luncheons appeared on our e-mail calendars, pocket PCs, and day planners as recurring Nordie's at Noon ("NaNoon") appointments. Like any group of young lunching women, we talked about our latest career moves, the men in our lives and, if we had them, our children and their escapades. But unlike other women our age, our conversations eventually turned to more serious issues: issues our "non–breast cancer friends" could not have imagined.

Our NaNoon luncheons began as a party of two, Patti and Jana, who met each other at their oncology clinic while getting monthly infusions of chemotherapy. The two instantly became "chemo friends." After all, Patti was only twenty-four years old when she was diagnosed with breast cancer, and Jana was twenty-seven, so the two had a lot in common!

The duo became a trio after Jana ran into her high school acquaintance, Jen, at a breast cancer survivors' luncheon.

Incredibly, Jen, too, had been diagnosed with breast cancer at the age of twenty-seven.

Less than a year later, the party of three expanded to four, when Patti learned that her college sorority sister, Kim, was diagnosed with breast cancer at the age of thirty. Kim eagerly joined our monthly luncheons for the hope, camaraderie, and support they could provide.

Patti was the youngest in our group and our only singleton. Tall, athletic, and slim, she would stride into Nordie's wearing the latest in casual business wear. She always looked the very model of today's bright young career woman. As a consultant for a large IT firm, she kept her nose to the grindstone at work. But after work and at our lunches, her wide smile and humorous "Patti-isms" often had us laughing hysterically. Independent and determined, Patti lived life to its fullest and refused to let breast cancer slow her down. Her priorities were family, friends, church, and career; but right through her treatments, she continued her search for Mr. Right.

Jana, the oldest in this young group, was the first to be diagnosed. "Jana Banana," as we called her, packed a lot of energy in her five-foot-two-inch frame. She was all girl when it came to jewelry, purses, and shoes. On weekends, though, her tom-boy side emerged as she pursued her constant goal of "getting in shape." Jana talked incessantly, and never took herself too seriously. Yet she was always serious and committed to her profession as a clinical researcher and to her volunteer work. While juggling ideas for her upcoming wedding, she also became a "walking brochure" of facts and stats about breast cancer.

Tall and slender, Jen carried herself with a polished, classic style even while pregnant. She had a smile as wide as Julia

Roberts's and an upbeat sense of humor that saw the glass as "half full" in nearly every situation. The rest of us were in awe of the organized way she juggled multiple commitments to family, friends, career, church, and volunteer work. Her optimistic attitude, coupled with a willingness to listen, made her the kind of friend whom others treasure. It was only as we got to know her that she admitted to feeling a little off-balance sometimes as she tried hard to please everyone else in her life.

Kim was a whirlwind of energy; she had so much self-confidence that she looked as if she could run circles around any big-city woman. Actually, she was from a rural town and had married her high school sweetheart. We teased her about being chronically late, but it was only, she would protest, because there was much she wanted to accomplish. She called herself a "recovering attorney" who had left her law firm after cancer so that she could start her own public affairs and motivational speaking business through which she could empower others. She considered herself lucky to be pursuing work she felt truly passionate about. We called her our "sexy professional" because of her clothing style. Of all of the Nordie Girls, Kim was the most open and free in sharing her story and all its details.

So there we were—four women in our twenties and early thirties; each at a different phase of life when diagnosed, and each at a different stage of treatment when we met. But our common bond was ever present: a sense that life is a precious gift and that maybe our affliction was a blessing in disguise because it made us appreciate life all the more. Our time together at Nordie's was therapeutic. When no one else could possibly understand what it was like to walk around with a "fake boob" or to go through breast reconstruction, we were there for each other. A special sisterhood was formed, and we eagerly looked forward to our time together.

In addition to sharing a breast cancer diagnosis, we were extremely driven, compassionate women on a mission to educate others about our disease and to make a positive difference in thousands of lives. The cliché "If I help just one person by sharing my story . . ." was not acceptable to any of us. We wanted to do more. After getting to know one another as friends and becoming literal "bosom buddies," the idea for this book began to percolate. We had all been disappointed with the lack of information available to us as young women newly diagnosed with breast cancer, so we wanted to share our experiences. We felt that other young women and their friends and families could benefit from what we had learned. So, *Nordie's at Noon* was born.

In order to share each of our perspectives on our breast cancer journeys, every *Nordie's at Noon* chapter features an introductory discussion in the setting of a Nordie's luncheon, followed by our individual perspectives and personal stories.

It is our greatest desire that readers will be empowered to be proactive with their health and lives, and that they will realize what we were surprised to learn ourselves: No one is "too young" for breast cancer.

Patti, Jana, Jen, and Kim

CHAPTER ONE

Help, I Have a Lump!

— Nordie's Café —
June 2002

From the beginning, we had a favorite corner booth at the Nordstrom Café, or Nordie's, as we affectionately called it. Patti always arrived early, cake in hand, to claim our favorite spot, a booth that offered comfortable seating, a view of the café entrance, and a table large enough to hold salads, plates of chocolate mousse cake, our organizers and notebooks, and the four of us. Jen arrived next, and would find Patti cheerfully devouring her chocolate mousse cake before her food order arrived. By the time Jen returned with her tomato-basil soup and salad, Jana had arrived. In the meantime, Kim would usually call Patti to say, "I'll be a little late." Just as the server brought Jana her food, Kim would dash in and order her salad and the pasta special. We quickly settled into a routine and rarely deviated from our usual food choices or order of arrival.

After some brief chatter from Patti about a cute guy at work, it was time to hear about the latest exploits of Kim's young son, Brandon. Then Jana chimed in with an update on her business travels, and Jen reminded us about the great shoe sale downstairs.

Once we had decided to write a book together, Patti assumed the role of secretary, keeping her laptop handy to take notes. Jen became the overall organizer, keeping the rest of us on track, and Kim, who had made many connections through her community work, would play a more prominent role when it came time to promote the book. Finally, Jana's job was to make sure that some fun was interspersed with all the work. She insisted we celebrate milestones with pedicures and gifts.

On this particular day, we tried to make sense of how each of us had felt when we discovered our respective lumps.

"Let's call our first chapter 'Help! I have a lump,'" suggested Jen.

Jana turned jokingly to Patti: "Maybe we should call it 'Finding Martha the Milk Dud.'"

Once, during a TV news interview, Patti had compared her lump to a Milk Dud, affectionately referring to it as "Martha the Milk Dud." "I'll never forget that quote," said Kim, and we all chuckled. We hadn't lost our sense of humor.

As we left to go back to work, each of us was thinking about The Day: the day each one of us found her lump.

Patti

It started when I was soaping up in the shower one day . . . honest, that's how I found my lump. My family has a long-standing history of breast cancer, but all my relatives were postmenopausal when they were diagnosed. In the fall of 1998, I was twenty-four years old and preparing to be in the weddings of two of my best friends, Donna and Dione. The weddings were only three weeks apart, and I was excited about both of them. Breast cancer was the last thing on my mind.

Recently, I'd gone from working two jobs and just getting by to securing a job at an international consulting firm. Finally, I could afford real Kraft Macaroni and Cheese, and I didn't have to juggle to pay my bills each month. All was going according to my plan.

I was born Patricia Susan Balwanz in Pittsburgh, Pennsylvania, soon after my dad came back from Vietnam. My father was a nuclear engineer and my mother a microbiologist. Eventually, something or "Someone" spoke to my dad, because after my brother, David, was born, our family moved to Richmond, Virginia. There, my father pursued his doctor of ministry degree and my mother stayed home to take care of David and me. From Virginia we moved to Farber, Missouri, where my dad served as minister for the Farber and Mt. Olivet Presbyterian Churches.

When I was in sixth grade, our family moved to Columbia, Missouri, so that my mom could pursue a degree in physical therapy, and David and I could have a "big-city" education. After junior high, I headed off to high school to become a Hickman Kewpie. That's right; my school was the only high school in the country that had chosen a naked baby doll for its mascot! I've always loved sports, and I represented our beloved Kewps on the swimming, diving, volleyball, softball, and basketball teams. I even earned Columbia's "Athlete of the Week" honor during my senior year.

In 1992, I enrolled at Southwest Missouri State University in Springfield, Missouri. During rush, I joined the Alpha Sigma Alpha (ASA) sorority. At first, I wasn't sure about sororities, and I thought about de-pledging almost every day for the first three months. But as time passed I grew to love sorority life; ultimately, I was nominated for Greek Woman of the Year. It was during our hectic sorority pledge week that I met Dione, a fellow pledge who became one of my best friends.

My college summers were spent working as a pool lifeguard in Columbia during the day and breaking into the same pools after hours for midnight swims with friends. That's how I met Donna, a fellow lifeguard who became my summer confidante, and eventually a lifelong friend.

For nearly two years after college graduation, I worked as a leadership consultant for my sorority; my job entailed traveling around the country and visiting college chapters of ASA. Then I returned to Missouri and rented an apartment down the road from my grandmother in Kansas City. When I landed my information technology consulting job, I felt that my career was taking off. Life was good.

Health insurance came with my new job, so I decided it was time for that all-important "yearly exam." I couldn't get an appointment for three months for a yearly physical, but asked whether I might get my breast checked sooner because I'd found a strange lump. "I have a history of fibrocystic lumpiness in my breast tissue, but this lump is different," I said.

The response was immediate. "Of course. How about seeing the nurse practitioner . . . tomorrow?"

So the next day, there I was, getting felt up by a nurse practitioner. The lump wasn't consistent with what she had felt before in cancerous breasts, but because of my family history, she arranged for me to have a baseline mammogram and ultrasound scan the next week. I got used to that sentence because I heard it again and again during the next four appointments: "It's not consistent with a cancerous breast, but because of your family history, we'll send you to the next step."

The next step was a biopsy. My grandmother went with me for my outpatient surgery. We weren't sure what to expect, but we knew the basics: needles, cuts, and a shipment of my breast tissue to the Mayo Clinic for evaluation. I knew in my heart that it was not going to be good news. When I stayed with my then boyfriend, Ben, the night before the biopsy, he felt the lump, and he agreed: In the month since I had found the lump, it had changed and gotten bigger. I cried myself to sleep that night in Ben's arms.

Jana

I was lost in the story of Michael Crichton's *Airframe* when the airplane began to shake and pitch violently, dropping thousands of feet in the air. At the same time, on an airplane myself, I felt a pain in my left breast, so sharp that it took my breath away. In an instant, I was brought back to reality, and I looked up from my book. Taking a deep breath to calm myself, I gazed out the window. I was relieved when the pain subsided.

I was fine for the rest of the flight from Kansas City to Tucson, and my mind wandered. I considered the birthday I had celebrated a few months ago, and how turning twenty-seven had officially catapulted me into my "upper twenties." I smiled as I imagined my forthcoming marriage to Chris, who had asked me to marry him a few weeks earlier as we stood in front of one of Kansas City's famous fountains. He had pulled a stunning engagement ring out of the small fifth pocket in his jeans. As I studied the princess-cut diamond that now adorned my finger, I was filled with happiness as I dreamt about our future together.

At the same time, I admit that I felt a little nervous about settling down. After all, I was an independent career woman who had planned some day to live in a loft in a big city. I certainly had not planned to get married and live in a 1950s tract house in the Midwest.

Still, things seemed to be falling into place in my life. I was born in Colorado and lived there through tenth grade. Shortly after turning sixteen, I moved to Michigan to live with my dad and his new wife—my stepmom, Patti. My father was an officer in the U.S. Army, so, as an "army brat," I attended three high schools before finishing my junior and senior years in Lansing, Kansas.

Lansing was a culture shock. My graduating class had fewer than 130 students—compared to my previous school where my class had numbered nearly 1,000. But in this small town and small school, I was able to excel. And I met friends who are still close to me today. I didn't travel far to college, just down the road to the University of Kansas (KU), where I had a full-ride ROTC scholarship and pledged the Delta Delta Delta (Tri Delta) sorority. I spent two fun-filled years at KU before transferring to Washburn University in Topeka to complete my bachelor of science degree in nursing.

After a year as a charge nurse in a private hospital, I landed a job in corporate America as a clinical research associate. This job required that I travel around the country monitoring clinical drug trials, and despite a hectic schedule that earned me a lot of frequent flyer miles, I felt healthy and happy. If the frenetic pace left me exhausted sometimes, I counted it as good exhaustion, especially since I made sure to mix play with work.

Whatever city I found myself in, I always did something to enjoy myself after completing my job. In Southern California, I rented a convertible, put the top down, and cruised the Pacific Coast Highway at sunset. In New York City, I extended my stay into a long weekend so that I could attend the U.S. Open tennis finals. In Florida, I stayed at a beachfront hotel and let the surf spray my feet as I walked at the ocean's edge. In Colorado, I skied and visited old friends. Sometimes, Chris was able to join me on a traveling weekend, as he did in Seattle and later in San Francisco. We loved those romantic getaways.

After landing in Tucson, I slung my bag over my shoulder and started down the jet way. Suddenly, the sharp pain in my breast returned. So, instead of heading for the baggage claim, I detoured to the women's restroom. I secured myself behind the flimsy metal door of the bathroom stall and gently touched my left breast through my shirt. My fingers gravitated to the point of tenderness, and I immediately confirmed that the pain got sharper with touch. I did not feel a lump at that time, because I was not looking for one. "I'll check it again when I get to the hotel," I told myself.

In my hotel room, I performed a series of rather neurotic rituals that were the result of being a frequent business traveler: I inspected the sheets for cleanliness; made sure there were no bugs hiding in the closet; verified that the tub was hairless; made note of the number of doors between my room and the nearest stairwell in case of a fire; and finally ordered room service. Then, while waiting for my room service order, I performed a breast self-exam (BSE).

As a registered nurse, I knew how to perform a BSE properly. I began by looking at each breast. There was no visible lump or bump. No redness, swelling, or bruising. Next, I used my hand and in a "pie wedge" pattern began to feel my breast tissue. The pie wedge ensured that I wouldn't miss a spot. In the upper, outer quadrant of my left breast, I found it. A hard, palpable lump, about the size and shape of a lemon drop. And it hurt.

I showered, got dressed, and went to sit on the balcony of my hotel room. I wanted to enjoy the Tucson sunset and admire my engagement ring sparkling in the southwestern sun, but I couldn't focus on my ring, my wedding, or my room service order. Thoughts of the lemon-drop-sized lump I had just discovered tugged at my cheery thoughts and tainted the afternoon glow.

Once before, while in college, I'd discovered a lump. An ultrasound scan showed that the lump was a just a cyst. It had disappeared: Surely this one would, too. But that first lump wasn't painful, nor was it quite this prominent. And the first lump was in my right breast. This new lemon-drop lump was in my left breast. My brain and my nursing education said it was probably nothing, but gut instinct told me the lump was just not right. It should not be there.

As a nurse, I knew the prudent thing to do was monitor the lump through one menstrual cycle and schedule an appointment with my gynecologist in the next thirty days. So that is what I did. During the next month, I compulsively monitored the lump. Nearly every time I had a moment of privacy, I would feel to see whether it was still there. I knew it was, because at times it was still painful. But I would check anyway—in the shower, while lying in bed right before falling asleep, and again when I woke up in the morning. I began each day by hoping the lump would not be there. But it did not disappear.

The lump interfered with my wedding planning. I was scheduled to be married in a mere five months, and I was "supposed" to focus on that. But it was hard to live up to the spirit of the adage "Enjoy the wedding planning—this is the fun part!" One day, during my quest for the perfect wedding gown, a bridal salon attendant explained that I would not have my dress fitted until a few weeks before my wedding. When I asked why, she explained, "You never know—you could gain weight in the next few months, or even get sick and lose weight. Then alterations would have to be done all over again." I swallowed hard. Were her words a premonition of what was to come?

When I told Chris about my appointment with my gynecologist, he was not overly concerned, nor was he even after I had him feel the lump. My gynecologist, too, told me that it didn't "feel like cancer," that it was probably nothing. Besides, I was "too young for breast cancer." But I was still worried, so I asked my gynecologist to refer me to a surgeon for an evaluation. I wanted to be certain that this lump really was "nothing." The surgeon, too, told me that at my age, it was highly unlikely my lump was cancerous. But to be sure, she suggested an open biopsy, which meant outpatient surgery to remove the entire lump under local anesthetic.

To accommodate my travel, we scheduled the biopsy for a few weeks later. By now, Chris was becoming slightly more concerned, though he tried to get me to stop worrying that it was cancer. When I insisted the lump could be cancerous, he reminded me that I had researched breast biopsies and had found that 80 percent of the test results were negative. But I reminded Chris that my grandmother had died of breast cancer when I was young and that his grandmother had died of breast cancer when he was young.

With the biopsy scheduled, I felt I should tell my parents and a few close friends. On the way home from selecting my wedding flowers, I told my stepmom. She was instantly worried. The few friends I told were also concerned, but not scared. They thought the biopsy would prove my lump was not cancerous.

Meanwhile, as fate would have it, I was assigned to work on a prostate cancer study. One night in my hotel room, I tried to enjoy a $20 cheeseburger with cold fries; but as I sat staring at a blue mini-carnation in a bud vase on the room-service tray, I thought about the cancer patients in the drug study and how sorry I felt for them. I had read their cases and had followed them via their medical reports and the handwritten, hardly legible progress notes. I'd read about their reactions, the shock they had shown to their diagnoses of cancer, and about the severe pain as the cancer metastasized to their bones. I even read about one patient who had died from his cancer.

That night, during my daily phone call home to Chris, I began to cry when I described the cancer study. Actually, sob is more like it. I just sobbed. Chris asked me what was wrong and whether I wanted to talk about it. But how could I explain to the love of my life that I was crying because of my own fear and my continuing gut feeling that the lump in my breast was cancerous? Though I had already told him I thought it was cancer, the feeling was much stronger that night. I felt so lonely after I hung up. As I cried myself to sleep in one corner of the king-sized bed, I wondered how it would feel to have cancer and to know you could die from it.

In hindsight, my involvement in the prostate cancer study helped prepare me for my own eventual cancer diagnosis. Reading the medical charts provided a crash course in Cancer Terminology 101, which was very useful later when I needed to ask the right questions and understand the answers related to my own disease. Having knowledge about my health situation and options were vital in helping me cope with my diagnosis.

Jen

I will never forget the day I found my lump. It was a cold November morning in 1999, and I was in the shower looking at my growing, pregnant belly. I was thrilled to be expecting my first child, and I was thoroughly enjoying pregnancy. But as I performed my monthly breast self-exam, a shiver went through my body. I felt a "rock" in my left breast.

When I asked my husband, Matt, to feel my breast, he felt the lump, too. I had an appointment with my obstetrician the following week, so I waited until then to bring it up; but from the moment I felt the rock, I worried. Whatever it was, I knew it should not be there.

For the most part, my life had been very much like "Leave-It-To-Beaver-Cleaver," as my husband liked to say. I grew up as an only child in a loving family. Because of my father's military career, we lived overseas and all around the United States. By the time I was twenty-one, I had seen more places than most people see in a lifetime. My mom, Kaki, was a teacher before I was born, but she stayed home to raise me until I entered high school. My dad, Jim, was busy with his career as a military officer, but he was always there for us. To this day, my parents continue to be two of the most influential people in my life.

Music and dance were my biggest passions when I was growing up. I can still see myself as a little girl dancing and singing on our coffee table. I loved to perform, and I took every kind of dance class—from toe to tap—until middle school. Then I moved from dance to choir, which remained a big part of my life through college. In fact, music serves as the soundtrack of my life. I can hear an old song and remember exactly what I was doing in my life when that song was popular.

Like Jana, I, too, lived in Lansing, Kansas. I moved there in time for my freshman year of high school. A lot of the other kids had gone to school together since kindergarten, so they were a tight-knit bunch. It wasn't easy to break in. I still have a few close friends from high school, but I don't think of that time as the "glory days."

College was different. I relished the freedom to be on my own, to come and go as I pleased. It was easy to make friends because my school was small. In my freshman year, I joined the Zeta Tau Alpha sorority (ZTA), and I found an amazing group of young women who were there for me no matter what. I went from being an only child to living with fifty "sisters," and although it took some adjusting, I loved every minute of it. To this day, a group of ZTA sisters and I meet for dinner every so often; and for one weekend a year, we escape our busy lives as wives, mothers, and working women to take an overnight trip together.

I believe that, in addition to helping me receive an excellent liberal arts education, God led me to Baker University in Baldwin, Kansas, for three important reasons: (1) to meet my future husband; (2) to become a member of ZTA so that I could make lifelong friends; and (3) to save my life.

The Susan G. Komen Breast Cancer Foundation (Komen), founded by Nancy Brinker in memory of her sister, Suzy, who died of breast cancer at the age of thirty-six, was adopted by ZTA as its national philanthropy during my junior year. The mission of the foundation is to eradicate breast cancer as a life-threatening disease by advancing research, education, screening, and treatment. Through my work with Komen, I became aware of the Three Steps to Early Detection:

- Annual mammography beginning at age forty
- Clinical breast examinations (a breast exam by a physician) at least every three years beginning at age twenty and annually after age forty
- Monthly breast self-examination beginning by age twenty

Without that knowledge, I don't think I would have been performing self-exams, and I shudder to think what the outcome could have been.

Matt and I spent our first two years of college as "friends." We would take each other to date parties when we didn't feel like taking a "real" date. During my junior year, I spent a semester at Harlaxton College in England—a wonderful time of studying and maturing. When I returned, Matt and I decided to "try" dating, even though both of us were nervous about possibly ruining a good friendship. We fell in love and, two years later, in 1995, we married.

One of the best things about falling in love with your best friend is that he already knows your faults, and despite that, he still loves you. Matt accepted that I'm so dedicated to order that I like the clothes in my closet and drawers arranged by color. I accepted the fact that my more laid-back husband leaves lights on and forgets to put his dishes in the dishwasher.

For the next four years, we were both busy with our careers—his as a high school teacher and basketball coach and mine in marketing for a large telecommunications company. But in 1999, we decided to start a family; soon after, I found out I was pregnant.

Six weeks later, I handed out roses to breast cancer survivors as a volunteer at the Komen Race for the Cure. I was feeling a little queasy from the pregnancy, and I was not excited about going to the 6:00 A.M. event. But when I saw all the women, I was overcome with emotion. One young woman in a pink survivor shirt pushed a baby stroller across the finish line. I was amazed that someone so young could have had breast cancer. Like many others, I had always assumed it was an older woman's disease. God surely sent me there that day because, later, remembering that sea of pink survivor shirts helped me believe I could beat this disease.

In October, my P.E.O. (a women's philanthropic educational organization) chapter offered a program on breast cancer because October is Breast Cancer Awareness Month. One of our members passed around a breast form, which is similar to the equipment women use to increase breast size, and asked us to feel how many lumps were in it. As she went through the risk factors for breast cancer, I made a mental checklist and was pleased to find that I had none of the risk factors. No woman on either side of my family had been diagnosed; I was not a heavy drinker, nor was I overweight; I was healthy, and pregnant, before age thirty. I was amazed, though, at how many lumps in the breast form I did not find. I felt only three, but there were seven. Each one felt different. Some were round like marbles, whereas others had sharp edges like a diamond. After missing so many lumps in the breast form, I know I pressed a little harder in my own self-exams, and that probably helped me find my tumor.

When I saw my obstetrician the week after I discovered the lump, she told me the baby was progressing nicely, and we were both happy about that. But when I told her about finding a lump, she gave me a breast exam and then immediately ordered a sonogram. If the lump was a cyst, we would leave it alone for now, she said, and if it was something else, we would treat it. I am grateful for my doctor's persistence since I was pregnant, otherwise healthy, and had no family history of breast cancer; but her concern scared me.

Matt was teaching, so I couldn't call him, but as soon as I returned to work, I phoned my mom and burst into tears. I was so afraid that I could hardly catch my breath. My mom kept saying, "Jen, don't worry. It's probably a benign cyst. Your obstetrician is just being super-careful." But I still felt afraid.

Matt was coaching basketball at school, and his schedule was swamped, so my mom went with me to the sonogram appointment just a few days later. She had made grand plans for us to go shopping for maternity clothes afterwards.

I asked the technician what we were looking for on the screen, and she explained that if the lump were a cyst, we would see fluid. I asked whether she saw any fluid. Instead of answering, she went to get the radiologist, and my heart hammered with fear. The radiologist ordered a mammogram. I was promised that my baby would be shielded from the x-rays, but it was important that we do this. Now. We cancelled our shopping plans.

The mammogram revealed something much smaller than what the sonogram had shown, but a surgical opinion was necessary. I was thankful that the surgeon I was referred to was able to fit me in the following day. He agreed that whatever it was, it needed to come out.

A biopsy was scheduled for the next day, a Thursday. The procedure itself was a breeze. I've had menstrual cramps that felt worse, but I was terribly frightened about the effect of all this on our baby. We didn't learn the results until Monday, and it was the longest weekend of my life. Matt tried to keep me busy, but all I could think about was the possibility of having cancer.

How could something as wonderful as a baby and as awful as cancer be growing in my body at the same time?

Kim

It was a cold, dreary Saturday in January, a typical Midwestern winter day. My husband, Scott, and I were planning our son's second birthday party. Brandon was our first child, and we wanted everything to be special. On his first birthday, Brandon hadn't known quite what to expect, but this year I was sure he would be the life of the party. He reminded me of the Energizer Bunny—going and going and going. I couldn't wait to see the look in his eyes when he blew out his candles and opened his gifts. I lived for such moments.

On Brandon's first birthday, Scott and I had started a tradition of having two parties—one for our many friends in town and one for family members, most of whom lived in Hallsville, the small town in Missouri where I grew up. As a party theme I'd chosen the "Year of Elmo" because Brandon was mesmerized by the movie *Elmo in Grouchland;* he would walk around the house and chant, "Elmo loves you, Elmo loves you." On this particular Saturday, I was a pretty typical crazed mom trying to meet my self-imposed deadlines for getting out party invitations.

Scott and I were living out our dreams. We both grew up in rural mid-Missouri and were high school sweethearts. We were also the first persons in each of our families to go to college and leave our small towns. We married after college, right before I started law school. After I completed law school, Scott, after a stint in corporate America, pursued his lifelong dream of becoming a firefighter.

I practiced law for a brief period after law school, and then went to work as director of community affairs for the mayor of Kansas City, Missouri. I also ran a good friend's campaign for city council and, when he won, went to work as his senior policy advisor. Now I was heading up an urban revitalization project. Both Scott and I believed we were making a difference in our community. Our careers were on track, we were the parents of a healthy, beautiful son, we were still deeply in love, and our dreams of the future included planning many more of Brandon's birthday parties.

But as I put together party invitations, I remembered it was the fifth day of the month and time to perform my monthly BSE, something I'd been doing faithfully ever since Patti—my sorority sister and coauthor of this book—was diagnosed with breast cancer.

I went into my bedroom and started the ritual of feeling my breasts; first, while lying down, then while standing in front of the mirror to visualize changes. I was in such a hurry that I shortened the exam, doing it only in front of the mirror. I stood with my arms at my sides and looked for changes in each breast. No changes. Then I raised my hands above my head . . . nope. No change. I pressed my hands firmly against my hips and flexed my chest muscles . . . again, no changes. No dimpling, redness, or swelling, and no changes in the nipple. I even went further and gently squeezed each nipple to see whether there was discharge. They were clean. Then, keeping my fingers flat, I moved in a circular, spiraling motion from underarm to collar-bone to the bra-line bottom of my left breast. No lumps or thickening. Everything seemed normal.

However, in my right breast, I felt something different—a lump the size of a golf ball, large and palpable. I hadn't felt this lump the month before when I had performed my BSE. How could it have grown this size in merely one month? It didn't hurt, but Patti's breast cancer diagnosis made me immediately fear the worst. Scott felt the lump, too, and since I performed regular BSEs and knew how my breasts felt normally, and hadn't felt the lump the month before, he agreed that I should see a doctor.

It was the weekend, so I had to wait two long days before making an appointment. I tried to think positively. Many women have fibroid cysts, I reminded myself, and the statistics say that eight out of ten breast lumps are not cancerous. Breast lumps are very common before menopause, and they usually go away by the end of the menstrual cycle.

However, I also knew that you should never ignore a change in your breast. Over the next two days, I felt my breast every hour or two to see whether the lump had gone away. But it was always there. On Monday, the doctor felt it, too, but was reas-suring. Given my age and with no family history of breast cancer, it probably was just a cyst. Still, a mammogram would make sure. Mammograms aren't recommended until women reach forty because the dense breast tissue in younger women make it difficult to read the films, so I'd never had one before. But soon I was sitting with my bra and shirt off, wearing a thin paper gown and waiting to get my breasts smashed. At least that's what it looked like. I wondered what type of man could have invented this machine. Actually, the mammogram was more of a pinch than a smash.

Because my breast tissue was so dense, an ultrasound scan followed. After looking at both reports, the radiologist recommended a surgical biopsy "just to be safe." My appointment was set up for three days later.

By now, I was more than a little scared, even though everyone kept saying, "You're young, healthy, and have no family history. It's probably nothing."

But it hadn't been "nothing" in Patti's case, and she was only twenty-four. Also, after doing research, I found that more than 85 percent of breast cancer patients have no family history of the disease. I thought about Brandon, and the birthday party we were planning. I wanted to be there for his third birthday, his fourth birthday, his first day of kindergarten . . .

After the appointment, I decided to let my family and a few close friends know what was going on. I called Patti and asked her what I should expect. I'm glad I made that call. She comforted me and helped put my mind at ease.

Two weeks after I had first felt my lump, I had a biopsy. My right breast was marked with a marker, I was given a local anesthetic, and before I knew it the biopsy was over. I tried to take comfort in knowing that Scott and my parents were there with me. I would learn the results in a week.

As I waited, I tried not to think about cancer. My stitches seemed to be healing fine, and from the outside, my breast looked normal, except for the two-inch surgical scar. I felt fine. Next Friday, I thought, I'll have my stitches removed and life will go on as before.

That's what I told myself.

D-Day
(Diagnosis Day)

— Nordie's Café —
July 2002

*W*e arrived at Nordie's in our usual order, Kim beaming as she said, "On time today!" Jana was in high spirits because she and Chris were about to take a much-needed vacation. Patti excitedly shared her recent computed tomography (CT) scan test results: "Everything looked stable with no signs of new cancer!" Jen accepted compliments on her new haircut, and then steered the conversation to our book. Today the topic was "Diagnosis Day," what we more commonly refer to as our "D-Day."

As they had from day one, Jana and Patti went to the same surgeon and medical oncologist. "Our surgeon has a heart of gold," said Patti. "I knew when I met her that she puts her patients first and keeps up with all the latest research." Jana nodded in agreement. Patti and Jana also shared monthly infusion treatments at the chemotherapy clinic. While they compared notes, Kim and Jen shared their experiences with different surgeons and medical oncologists. We talked about the way we felt during our first few office visits, and how we disliked the thin paper gowns we had to wear, and how frustrating it was to read the same outdated magazines in the waiting room week after week.

The sounds of the café blended into the background as we talked about the parade of procedures, tests, and visits from friends and family.

"How did you feel when you were told, 'You have breast cancer'?" asked Kim.

"Actually," Jen recalled, "I think it was harder to say the words 'I have breast cancer' than to hear them."

Jana and Patti recounted their 5:00 P.M. appointments. "You never want a five o'clock appointment," said Patti, "because it probably means you've got the big 'C' and there's a lot to discuss."

Instinctively, Patti had lowered her voice. Jana joked, "You'd think cancer was contagious the way we say the word in such a hushed tone." She glanced at the other tables in the restaurant. All of us wondered, How many other women at Nordie's were talking about breast cancer? How many had experienced their own D-Days?

Patti

One ultrasound scan, one mammogram, and one anesthesia-vomit-wracked biopsy later, I got "the call." Would I bring a family member with me for a 5:00 P.M. appointment on Friday? My dear friend Donna, just back from her honeymoon, said she would come, and so would Larkin, another friend.

At the doctor's office, I explained that my family lived out of town, so my two friends were with me as my family. The nurses, who all knew what the "Friday at five appointment" meant, offered sympathetic smiles.

A few minutes later, the surgeon began telling me what I had already figured out: I had breast cancer. There it was, laid out like cards in a poker game. Not a royal flush, but a crap hand. Donna, level-headed and practical as always, whipped out her day planner and asked about "treatment options." My other "family member," Larkin, began to cry and reached for my hand. I just sat there, dumbfounded.

Between tears, Larkin blurted, "Will she die?" The doctor reassured her she would do everything possible to prevent that from happening. Larkin cried harder. Donna started asking medical questions: "Did you get clean margins? What stage is the tumor? Does Patti need to begin radiation immediately? What about chemotherapy and scheduling a mastectomy?"

I couldn't speak. I couldn't cry.

Thankfully, I was surrounded by people I loved. They reacted the way I felt inside. Part of me wanted to cry, as I'm doing now, as I write this. Part of me wanted to plow through my options and begin making decisions. And part of me wanted to start the last couple months over in a different body, one not inhabited by the nonclean margin, Stage I, aggressive cancerous lump that I'd taken to calling "Martha, the Milk Dud." A month ago, I was lifting drinks at my friends' weddings, preparing to give yet another toast, and doing the "hustle" or the "electric slide." Now I was a part of that group of people with cancer.

As we left the doctor's office, Larkin grabbed my hand and asked if we could pray. If someone had taken a picture, I think that moment would be more symbolic than any other of that afternoon. Three young women, tear-stained, scared beyond belief, and with conviction beyond reason, moving into an unknown battle, and asking for help from the only Power that could give it to us.

Jana

My biopsy took place on a Tuesday morning in June, and although I was nervous before the procedure, I don't remember the biopsy itself. I do remember the ride home, though, when my stepmom informed me that the surgeon had told her she didn't think it was cancer, so we shouldn't worry. I said, "I'll stop worrying after I know the pathology results." It was a relief the day after the biopsy to look at my left breast and know the lemon-drop lump had gone. The two-inch incision and resulting scar would serve as a reminder, I thought, always to perform my BSEs.

Around 5:00 P.M. the next day, the phone rang. It was my surgeon's receptionist, who said the doctor wanted to see me. "When?" I asked. "Now," she replied.

Now? Why would a doctor want to see a patient so late in the day? I wondered. And then I knew. When the receptionist called again, seconds after I'd hung up, to ask me to bring someone with me, my fears were confirmed.

Although I had planned to see Chris and my parents that evening, I couldn't reach any of them, so—independent woman that I thought I was—I decided to go by myself. But as I pulled out of my garage, I thought, "Wait a minute, am I really going to get possibly the worst news of my life, *alone?*"

As God would have it, at the moment I pulled out of the garage, my dad drove up. As soon as I told him where I was headed, he said, "I'm going with you." As we drove, his voice held a pleading note. "I'm sure your doctor just wants to see how you are doing." As if to say, "Tell me that's all it is." But all month I'd had a gut feeling that the lemon-drop lump was cancerous, and in the surgeon's office a few minutes later, my suspicion was confirmed.

The surgeon sat on her round stool with wheels so she was at eye level with us. She spoke softly, almost in a whisper, but to me it felt like a scream. "Your pathology report has come back positive for cancer. Now let's figure out what we are going to do."

My dad reached for my hand, but I was afraid that if I gave in to that loving gesture, I would lose my composure. So, reflexively, I went into my defense mode: the logical, matter-of-fact nurse Jana.

I had brushed up on my medical oncology lingo while working on the prostate cancer study, and now it came in handy. We spoke at length about all the options, and I should have left the office armed with lots of facts and "what-if scenarios." But despite the two hours of intense discussion, only one thing really soaked in: I have cancer.

When my dad and I walked into my house after meeting with my surgeon, Chris and Patti, my stepmom, were waiting with wide, glassy eyes and tear-stained cheeks. The doctor had called them while my dad and I were driving home. Both rushed to embrace me. Out of the blue, I said, "I need a cigarette!" Chris looked at me blankly because I'd given up smoking years earlier. Patti said, "Let's go get her a pack!" My dad said firmly, "Absolutely not!" Looking back on it, I realize that the entire exchange was odd. But at that moment, I was so helpless; I didn't know what else to say.

My parents left so that Chris and I could have some time alone. Immediately, I said, "I'll understand if you don't want to marry me now. I don't want you to go through this. I'm so sorry."

Chris looked dumbfounded. "Of course, I still want to marry you. We'll get through this together!" So we held each other, cried, and prayed silently that everything would be okay.

After our tears dried, Chris said he was hungry, so we went out to get something to eat. The sky had darkened as if for rain, only I don't remember any rain clouds. Then I saw it. Painted across the sky was the most brilliant rainbow I had ever seen. "Look!" I exclaimed. The rainbow seemed like a message from God telling us to have hope in the face of the storm we were about to endure.

Jen

My biopsy results came on Monday, November 22, just three days before Thanksgiving. All morning I waited anxiously, even skipping my shower for fear I might miss the doctor's call. Matt had gone to work—I'd insisted—but he came home at noon, wanting to be with me. He was sitting on our stairs, and when the phone finally rang and he saw my face as I listened, his head dropped into his hands. He told me later that he felt completely helpless, as if his whole world were crumbling. I was twenty-seven years old, twenty-two weeks pregnant with my first child, and yes, said the doctor, I had breast cancer.

Matt and I held each other tightly. Then I called my mom. I'll never forget how hard it was to say out loud, "Mom, I have cancer." She immediately burst into tears.

"I'm going to fight this," I promised. "Don't give up on me."

My mom first called my dad, and then her boss, explaining that I had called and that she wouldn't be coming back to work that day. In a very sweet gesture, my mom's boss rushed over so that my mom wouldn't be alone before my dad arrived.

Next, Matt phoned his mom, Pam, who was caught totally off guard. He hadn't told her about the biopsy because he thought the lump would turn out to be benign. When she first heard his solemn voice, she thought something was wrong with the pregnancy. He assured her that the baby was fine, and then proceeded to tell her that I'd been diagnosed with breast cancer. She, too, began to cry.

At the doctor's office, I had the eerie sensation of being outside myself, unable to believe this was really happening. To me. Yet both of my grandfathers, as well as an uncle and a great-grandfather, had lost their lives to cancer.

The doctor perched on a corner of his desk, and in a forthright way began giving details to Matt, my parents, and me. My cancer was invasive ductal carcinoma, meaning it had started in a milk duct and spread outside. The tumor measured 3.5 centimeters, about the size of a grape: not small, but not unusually large, either.

"Are you sure Jen has cancer?" my dad asked. "Could there have been a mix-up in the lab?" The doctor shook his head. "I'm sorry. We are sure."

When I went on to ask about our baby, his tone was comforting. He would take care of me, and my obstetrician would take care of the baby. Without a healthy mom, he reminded me, our baby didn't stand a chance. I remembered all of those pink shirts I'd seen at the Race for the Cure. There are more than two million breast cancer survivors today, I reminded myself. I can beat this. I will beat it for our baby's sake. I still wasn't sure how I could be treated for cancer while pregnant; but I was going to listen closely to what the doctors said, and I would also do research on my own. Nothing was going to stop me from bringing a healthy child into the world.

Matt told me later that when he first heard the diagnosis, he felt sure he was going to lose me and the baby; but after our doctor talked to us, he felt encouraged about what lay ahead.

As for me, I was still scared, but ready to fight.

Kim

A week after my biopsy, when I still hadn't heard from my surgeon, I began feeling hopeful. I figured "no news is good news." But when I went to have my stitches removed, the first thing the doctor said was "I have bad news. You have breast cancer." Four simple but life-altering words. Scott grabbed my hand as I fought back the tears. The biopsy results showed a cancerous lump that measured 4 by 3 centimeters. Matter-of-factly, the surgeon explained that I had two options: a mastectomy or a lumpectomy. He briefly explained what each entailed and said that his office would make appointments for me with an oncologist, a radiologist, and a plastic surgeon to help determine the proper course of treatment. As he spoke, I saw his mouth move, but I couldn't seem to hear his words. I was numb and in shock. "How could this be happening?"

Then my law school training kicked in, and I started barraging him with questions. What stage was my cancer? What type was it? How aggressive? If I were his wife or mother, what advice would he give? Patti had told me that building your "team" of doctors was important and that I should be my own advocate.

Okay. I had successfully run political campaigns; now we were talking about my life. I'd run a successful campaign here, too.

But the doctor's answers were short and curt. He reiterated my two surgical choices, but didn't answer my other pointed questions. That's when I decided to get a second opinion—and a new surgeon.

As soon as we left the doctor's office, I called Patti on my cell phone to tell her my diagnosis and to get her recommendation for a new doctor. I wasn't going to fight for my life with a surgeon who was impersonal, nonemotional, and noninformative. When she heard my news, Patti grew very quiet. Then, in typical Patti style, she said, "Welcome to the club!" We both laughed, although I wondered, "What are the odds that two good friends would both get breast cancer by the age of thirty?"

Once Scott and I left the doctor's office, I immediately did what every mother would do—I picked up Brandon from preschool. In the car, I held my little boy and cried. I kept thinking—I don't want to die. I want to see Brandon graduate from high school and college, get married, have children, and pursue his dreams. I want him to know his mother.

That evening, I made phone calls, first to my parents, then to close friends. Friday is my dad's poker night, so I talked to my mom. She started asking all kinds of questions, many of which I couldn't answer. I was my parents' only daughter, the youngest of their three children, and my mom and dad felt helpless; their baby had cancer and they were two hours away. My friends reacted in one of two ways: hysterical crying or absolute silence. It was so difficult and emotionally exhausting that finally Scott took over and sent out e-mails.

Even though my phone calls had exhausted me—or maybe because of that—I decided to attend a going-away party for a friend who was moving out of town to work on a U.S. Senate re-election campaign. Politics is a passion of mine, and I thought the party would let me escape the reality of my recent diagnosis. But as the evening wore on, the realization that I had breast cancer began sinking in; eventually, I became physically ill. I continued throwing up into the wee hours of the morning.

The uncertainty of what lay ahead and the fact that I didn't yet have a plan of attack against this killer that had invaded my body didn't sit well with my type-A, anal-retentive personality. Here I was, thirty years old, the mother of a soon-to-be two-year-old, and I'd just been diagnosed with breast cancer. Now what?

CHAPTER THREE

Choices, Choices, Choices

— Nordie's Café —
August 2002

Patti's meeting had run late, so our coveted corner booth was already taken when she arrived at Nordie's. Although this threw a kink in our lunchtime routine, we soon got our lunches, found a table, and began to catch up on each other's lives.

Patti told us about a cute guy at work ("But he has so much growing up to do!") and revealed her secret crush on one of her best "guy" friends. She wasn't sure whether their friendship could turn into something more. Jen offered encouragement, having married her best "guy" friend from college.

When the conversation turned to Jana, she commented that she was ready for her next hormone shot—her hormones were out of whack and she was eating dessert in addition to her usual ham-and-cheese panini. Patti, who was undergoing the same medical treatment, knew exactly what Jana was talking about.

Conversation soon steered to our book. Today, we were discussing the next chapter on treatment options. Jana suggested we call it "Choices, Choices, Choices." The rest of us nodded, recalling the countless medical appointments we kept while making decisions about treatment options.

"Understanding the pathology report was really hard," said Kim. Even Jana, a nurse and the designated medical expert of our group, admitted that she found the reports difficult to read, but for a different reason. She knew too much about how the information might impact her survival. "Sometimes," she said, "knowing too much adds fear, but I think it also helped me understand which questions to ask."

Kim was diagnosed a few years after the rest of us, so medical advances had brought her different treatment options. Jana, Patti, and Jen underwent surgery first, but Kim received chemotherapy before surgery. We were happy to learn about the progression of breast cancer research and the movement in the direction of finding a cure.

Although all of us shared the same disease, there were obvious differences: Our personalities, our lifestyles, our careers, and even our clothing styles were different. So as unique individuals we made different choices. In spite of our differences, we had similarities that went beyond breast cancer, including a common understanding of the importance of pedicures, men, and vacations. On a more serious note, we all shared a strong sense of hope and faith.

Against a backdrop of differences and similarities, we each made choices that were the best for us as individuals. And despite our varying treatment paths, we shared one choice: We chose to face breast cancer head-on, to fight it with all our might, and we were willing to do whatever it might take to live.

Patti

When initially diagnosed, I had an overwhelming number of choices to make. What surgery will I need? What pre- or posttreatment chemotherapy? Whom should I tell about my experience? Each choice would affect my future, my lifestyle, and my chances for recurrence.

The best piece of advice I received was this: "Contrary to what may be popular belief, everyone experiences cancer differently, so allow yourself to experience cancer your way."

My way included opting for a mastectomy, whereby the entire breast is removed, followed by a full TRAM (transverse rectus abdominis muscle) reconstruction. The surgeon would perform what I call a "cut and paste"—cutting the fat tissue from my abdomen and using it to form a new breast to paste in place of the old one. My reasons for these choices? I looked at cancer as a disruption in my life, and I wanted to return as quickly as possible to what I considered normal. A mastectomy meant not having to worry about the remaining breast tissue and the potential spread of disease to that tissue.

As for electing TRAM reconstruction, I attribute most of it to vanity. I figured that if I had to give up my natural breast, why not come out ahead with two nicely shaped ones (I could have the other one "reduced" for symmetry) and a flat stomach that would last until childbirth. One year later, I was wearing a two-piece swimsuit for the first time in my life.

Now if I had stopped there, this would be a short chapter. But there's more to it. Certainly the choices about initial treatment are important; I don't want to belittle their worth. But there were far greater decisions I made when diagnosed with cancer. And they had little relation to treatment options or the fact that I would likely be shiny and bald-headed in a matter of weeks.

First of all, whom should I tell?

After my close family and friends were aware of my diagnosis, I pulled out my address book and started making phone calls, alphabetically. A tough call was the one to my brother, who was serving with the Peace Corps in rural Africa. Tough because he wasn't in the United States with the rest of us, and tough because it was challenging to get my message to him along the dusty roads of Malawi. There were also some phone calls I couldn't make, mostly because I was scared of what I would say. My parents helped out with some of those calls and the others were just conversations that I had to have, some-times months after my diagnosis.

Looking back, rather than going alphabetically through my address book, I realize I would have benefited from deciding at the outset whom I would keep intimately involved in my experience.

But even more important than any of these decisions, I made the choice to live (a.k.a. "beat the cancer"). After diag-nosis, I was filled with a fighting spirit greater than the one that I had during those gut-wrenching basketball practices when our coach would ask, "Who wants to get on the line and sprint one more time?" Each time, I lined up for that one last sprint exercise.

No matter how tired I was, no matter how much easier it would have been to get a drink of water and sit down on the bench, I knew that if I ran "one more time," I'd be better off in the long run. That lesson stuck with me, and I used it when I was asked to find my "will to live." So following my diagnosis, I strapped on my tennis shoes and put my nose to the grind-stone (while stuffing Kleenex up it to stop the bleeding).

Those were the choices I made. Other choices were yet to come, but for now—cancer wasn't going to beat me; I was up at the line again.

Jana

After I was told I had breast cancer, my thoughts were thrown into a blender on high speed, and they went much like this:

Everythingallofthesuddenmovesatanincrediblepaceand
thoughtsarescrambledandthingsareconfusingandthings
flythroughyourmindandbackoutfasterthanyoucaneven
processthethoughtsandthenitallboilsdowntoonething
andtheworldseemstostop.

And although the world seemed to stop, my thoughts did not. I have cancer. I have no control over my body. It has betrayed me. I have cancer. I fed my body healthy foods, and even exercised regularly. I have cancer. I fed my body unhealthy fast foods and smoked cigarettes when I was a teenager and drank too much caffeine. I have cancer. I am helpless. I am scared. I am worried. I have cancer. I am supposed to get married in four months. I cannot get married—I am damaged. I am going to die. I have cancer. Am I going to die? I have a million things to do before I die. How long will I live? Do I need chemotherapy? I have cancer. Will I need surgery? A mastectomy? With reconstruction? Without reconstruction? Bilateral or unilateral? I have cancer. Implants? Saline or silicone? TRAM flap reconstruction? From my abdomen or from my back? Will I lose my hair? Will I throw up? Will I lose weight? Or get fat? I have cancer. Do I need radiation? A lumpectomy? Eastern medicine? I have cancer. Tijuana—I can get treatment there. Alternative medicine. I have cancer. Work. Sick leave. Vacation. I have cancer. Shit.

For the next few weeks, my days were filled with the sheer terror of realizing that I have cancer. Then there were doctors' appointments, telephone calls, e-mails, flowers, cards, balloons, tears, Web sites, toll-free numbers, stories about strangers who also have breast cancer. I felt hopeless and out of control.

But one day, I suddenly had a new thought: I am not hopeless and out of control because I have choices to make. Choices about my cancer treatment and about my life. The choices I made were these:

- I choose not to be hopeless, but to be hopeful.
- Yes, I'm going to die, but not today.
- Yes, I have cancer, but today I am alive.
- I choose to live tomorrow, and the next day, too. There is really nothing to stop me from living the next weeks, months, and years except that I have cancer.
- I do need to take care of that. And I will.

So, in order to live, I chose what I thought had the best potential for keeping me alive. I chose to have breast conservation surgery, which meant the rest of my tumor would be surgically removed, and if "clean margins" were obtained, the rest of my breast would remain. However, I also decided that if the surgeon couldn't obtain "clean margins," I would have a unilateral modified radical mastectomy without reconstruction.

In lay terms, that means my left breast tissue would be removed, including several lymph nodes from under my left armpit. If any of the cancer had spread to the lymph nodes, there was an increased likelihood that it had spread outside of the breast (metastasized), which would impact other treatment options such as chemotherapy. I also chose a silicone prosthesis (a.k.a. "fake boob"), rather than have breast reconstruction should I need a mastectomy. A silicone prosthesis is a permanent breast form that can be slipped inside a bra or swimming suit and taken out each night.

I also chose to go through chemotherapy with Adriamycin and Cytoxan, even though I knew it meant I'd be sick and probably lose my hair. That seemed a small price to pay for my life. Most important, I chose to let God hold my heart, mind, and body in His hands, and have my faith carry me on its wings. And, finally, with Chris, I chose to have our wedding on the date we had originally planned—now just four months away.

My last choice? I needed to find a wig!

Jen

After my diagnosis, I was floored when my surgeon recommended a full mastectomy. Everything I'd read said that the majority of women were good candidates for a lumpectomy, the procedure by which the surgeon removes only the tumor and some normal tissue around it. I hadn't even considered a mastectomy as an option.

At that point, we didn't know whether the cancer had spread to my lymph nodes. Surgery would show that and allow a way to determine my true stage. There are four stages of breast cancer, each one depending on the size of the tumor and how far it has spread from the original site. Because my tumor was larger than 2 centimeters, I was at least an early Stage II, which is still considered early breast cancer.

Because of my pregnancy and the need for chemotherapy, my surgeon took my case to a "tumor board," which consisted of representatives from a range of cancer disciplines who met regularly to discuss individual cases and, if possible, improve care. After the tumor board met, I talked to a radiation oncologist and a medical oncologist.

The radiation oncologist said that if I chose a lumpectomy, I would need to follow up with thirty radiation treatments, five days a week for six weeks. It's not a painful procedure, although it can irritate the skin. The purpose of radiation after a lumpectomy is to eradicate stray cells that might remain in the breast. Since I couldn't have radiation while pregnant, I would have to wait until my baby was born, in four and a half months. The radiation oncologist was very genial and willing to explain things. But as I was leaving, he said, "I hope I don't see you again." He thought a mastectomy was my best option.

The medical oncologist said that because of my age and the aggressive nature of the tumor I would need chemotherapy no matter what the status of the lymph nodes. If my lymph nodes were free of cancer, I'd need four rounds of chemotherapy; if I had positive lymph nodes, I'd need eight rounds. Plus six weeks of radiation. So like it or not, mastectomy or lumpectomy, I could count on chemotherapy.

Treatment for breast cancer while pregnant is not common— only forty cases were listed in the national cancer registry at the time of my diagnosis. But if a pregnant or postpartum woman is going to get cancer, it will likely be cancer of the breast. It occurs in about one in three thousand pregnancies.

Among those cases in the registry, the good news was that all the babies were born healthy, although sometimes prematurely, and the prognosis of a Stage II pregnant woman compared to a

Stage II nonpregnant woman showed the same outcome. One difference was that pregnant women are often diagnosed at a later stage because breasts change during pregnancy, and nursing makes it harder to detect a lump.

My obstetrician reiterated what my surgeon had said. She would let the other doctors take care of me, and she would take care of my baby. I would make frequent visits to her and I would undergo extra sonograms and testing.

I'd been fearfully waiting for someone to tell me that I should terminate my pregnancy for health reasons, so I was immensely relieved by what my obstetrician said. I could not have terminated my pregnancy, and I felt fortunate that I was halfway through pregnancy when the cancer was discovered. At this stage, my baby had all his or her vital organs and just needed time to grow.

Matt and I agonized over which surgery to choose. For reasons of vanity, I didn't want to have my breast removed. You spend most of adolescence waiting for these things to start growing, and now, at twenty-seven, I'd have to lose one? But when we asked each doctor what he would recommend for his own wife or daughter in a similar situation, all said they would recommend a mastectomy.

The pressure to decide was the backdrop to Thanksgiving, which we spent with our families. I tried to be cheerful; but I kept thinking how I had waited all this time to have a child, that I was finally ready, but now I might not live to raise him or her. In the middle of dinner I had to excuse myself to the restroom so that I could cry.

My surgeon had talked with a mentor of his who also believed a mastectomy offered the best long-term chances for survival. The conclusion seemed obvious. I needed to sacrifice my breast for my long-term health and for our baby. I took a deep breath, said yes, and have never looked back.

Kim

The three weeks after my initial diagnosis and before my treatment began were the longest weeks of my life. First, I knew I needed a second opinion. I was not happy with my first surgeon. For starters, I thought he should have reviewed my pathology report with me, and when I asked his nurse why he hadn't, she said crisply that he thought it was the job of my oncologist. To me, that was simply shifting the burden to others.

I had tried to read the report on my own, but it was filled with medical jargon too difficult to really understand, and that ticked me off. Here I was, a well-educated thirty-year-old woman trying to learn about my own cancer from a report too dense to understand, yet my surgeon wouldn't take the time to explain it to me.

My days soon were filled with doctors' appointments. Clad only in thin gowns that wouldn't tie in the back, I sat in one cold examining room after another while I waited and waited for the next doctor to come and look at my breast. In the first week alone, with Scott by my side, I had a chest x-ray and a bone scan, and I met with an oncologist, a radiation oncologist, and a plastic surgeon.

I still wonder why doctors can't do their exams and allow patients to get dressed before talking instead of carrying on a fifteen-minute conversation while you're sitting there in a paper-like gown, which by now is gaping open.

It helped that Scott went with me to my appointments—not only for moral support but to provide another set of ears. I even took a tape recorder to my first few appointments, and I also wrote down my questions in advance so that I wouldn't forget any.

In addition to medical experts, I sought advice from other breast cancer survivors, asking them what choices they'd made and why. I quickly learned that no one's cancer is the same and that I had to decide, along with my team of doctors, what the best course of treatment was for my case. I felt so much pressure. This wasn't a game of chess. I couldn't afford to make any wrong moves. The stakes were too high. How would I know whether I was making the right choice?

My cancer was very aggressive, but because I'd caught it early by performing my monthly BSE, I had a better chance of beating it. The bone scan and chest x-ray showed that the cancer had not spread to my bones or chest, but the doctors couldn't tell about the lymph nodes without performing surgery.

My oncologist recommended neoadjuvant chemotherapy—chemo treatments before surgery—because my tumor was relatively large and aggressive, and the margins were not "clean" after my initial biopsy, when my tumor was removed.

Even though it was driving me crazy not to have a finalized plan of attack, I decided to wait until after Patti's surgeon could give me a second opinion. And if I liked her, I planned to switch surgeons. Over and over from cancer survivors I'd heard this: "It's important to build the right team of doctors and make sure they communicate on a regular basis."

In between appointments, I read everything I could about breast cancer. *Dr. Susan Love's Breast Book* provided clinical information, and books such as *The Feisty Woman's Breast Cancer Book* and *Bosom Buddies* helped me keep a sense of humor about what I was experiencing.

I also searched the Internet for hours, and was comforted to learn that breast cancer, when localized to the breast, has nearly a 95 percent five-year survival rate. Also, I spoke to dozens of women who had had "the experience." (The day I was diagnosed, I chose to use the word "experience" and not "disease." To me, "disease" has a negative connotation, and I needed to stay as positive as possible.)

I was amazed by how many people had been touched by this experience. Mothers, daughters, sisters, wives, neighbors, and friends. I was also encouraged by the number of women whose experience had taken place ten, fifteen, or twenty years ago without a recurrence. They gave me hope. At the same time, I was discouraged to learn that there is no "cure" for breast cancer and that approximately forty thousand women a year die from breast cancer. Even if you go fifteen years without a recurrence, medical journals say you are never considered "cured."

When I saw Patti's surgeon, she spent two hours with Scott and me, walking us through treatment options. I, too, got the 5:00 P.M. appointment. She reviewed my pathology report and explained every detail. I had invasive ductal carcinoma, my tumor size was 4 centimeters, and I was a Stage II, possibly a Stage III, patient, depending on whether I had lymph node involvement. My surgery options, based on the type of cancer I had, were a lumpectomy and radiation, a mastectomy alone, or a mastectomy with reconstruction.

Because of the size of my tumor, the fact that I did not have clean margins, the aggressive nature of my cancer, and my age, my surgeon and I decided that a lumpectomy was not the best option for me. I knew that if I underwent a mastectomy, I wanted some type of reconstruction. The surgeon helped me decide to have a mastectomy with TRAM flap reconstruction, a procedure in which the plastic surgeon takes fat from the abdomen and builds a new breast. I actually smiled as I thought: "I'll be getting a new boob and a tummy tuck out of the deal!"

Since my tumor was large and the cells were dividing and growing quickly, I also chose chemotherapy before surgery. After four treatments of chemotherapy, I would have a mastectomy with immediate TRAM flap reconstruction; then, depending on lymph node involvement, I would have another four rounds of chemo and/or radiation.

For a while, I felt a real loss of control as I made choices. All my life, I've been so organized, able to look at every decision to see where it fits into my overall plan. As Scott would say with a laugh, "Kim has her CD collection alphabetized and her sock drawer color-coded." Now I was learning one of life's lessons: Sometimes you are not in control. Sometimes you just need to have faith in God and believe that everything will turn out for the best.

It was especially hard when I looked at my precious son. For a split second, I'd think, "What if I don't beat this thing? Brandon is so little, he won't remember his mommy." Then I would snap out of it and tell myself, "*You will beat it!* And you're here right now, and that's what matters!"

y

CHAPTER FOUR

Surgery:
And Then There Was One

— Nordie's Café —
September 2002

The dim lighting, the clatter of plates, and the bustling service at Nordie's Café were beginning to feel like a second home to us. Jana navigated the maze of strollers, monstrous purses, and shopping bags to slide into our corner booth while Jen related that on a recent business trip she had coughed through an entire meeting. "It ended up being bronchitis, but it was so embarrassing," she said. We toasted Kim's eighth and final round of chemotherapy, and then we got down to business.

"In chapter 4, we should talk about our surgeries," suggested Jen. "You know, 'And Then There Was One.'" For all of us, it felt like "just yesterday" that we were being wheeled into our respective surgical rooms. Three of us had used the same surgeon and agreed with Jana's assessment: "She was so compassionate and calming." Because of her insurance plan, Jen used another surgeon, but she found him just as compassionate.

Patti, Jen, and Kim chose to undergo mastectomies. Patti and Kim opted for immediate reconstruction using a TRAM flap. Since Jen was pregnant, it was important to minimize her time under anesthesia, so reconstruction for her was not an option. Jana's surgery was planned as a lumpectomy, with a mastectomy scheduled if necessary. "I went under the knife, not knowing whether I would wake up with a breast or not," Jana recalled.

"I knew I was going in for a mastectomy," Jen said, "still, waking up with a large scar on my chest and no breast was a little overwhelming."

"I was so focused on getting rid of the cancer, I didn't think about what it might be like not to have a breast," said Jana. "I just wanted all of the cancer gone."

We acknowledged that emotional scars plagued each of us, although at varying degrees. And even with immediate breast reconstruction, there was still mourning for the breast that was gone.

Still, after talking about it through lunch, we agreed we would go through the same surgeries and make the same choices if we had to do it all over again. It was strangely comforting to know, in hindsight, that each of us had chosen the best surgical options for our individual situations and had no regrets.

Patti

My attitude before surgery was "Let's get this over quickly so I can get on with my life." First, though, my stomach, conditioned to being fat-free, needed to be fattened so that my surgeon would have enough fat for the TRAM flap reconstruction. For five weeks, I went on a Nutty Bar binge. I must admit that part was fun.

The night before surgery, my parents, some close friends, and I went out to eat together. I was touched that my mom and dad were there, but only later realized how important their presence was. I was also happy to see my friends, but below the surface, it scared me that everyone was making such a big deal of my surgery.

The next morning, I worried that my veins would roll when they stuck me with the IV needle. I told the nurse to make a good stick, and on the third try she succeeded. During pre-op, my dad and I talked while my mom got warm blankets to keep me comfortable. I was more relaxed than the night before because now that it was happening all I had to do was get anesthetized, lie on an operating table, and wake up with a new breast and a flat tummy.

Shortly before the surgery, the Lord's Prayer played over the loudspeaker. This comforted me. My dad and I talked some more, and then it was off to surgery.

I woke up and saw my friend and housemate, Stephanie, sitting beside my bed. She still laughs because, as drugged as I was, I managed to ask her, "How was your day?" The rest of that day is hazy. The hospital staff continuously checked my vital signs to make sure blood was flowing through my new breast. Once, my mom freaked out because the machine stopped registering a pulse, but it turned out to be malfunctioning equipment, which was quickly replaced.

By the next day, I was more alert and able to use a morphine clicky-button to keep pain to a minimum. The nurses continued to come in and out all day. My best friends Donna and Dione visited. Donna watched them drain me dry—three direct hits on a vein, but no blood. Dione, who had driven four hours to see me, brought me a bouncing Tigger. My surgeon likened me to a bouncing Tigger—and the image stayed with me throughout my treatment. Yes, I was going to bounce back!

When I went home from the hospital three days later, my stomach was painfully tight and my new breast hurt and felt weird. But I had a breast, and thus a new joie de vivre.

Over the next few months, the plastic surgeon created a nipple and tattooed an areola on my breast. For me, the tougher parts were sorting through my feelings about my new body and my feelings about my relationship with my boyfriend, Ben.

Ben stuck by me as much as I would let him. After the mastectomy, he held my hand while I was in the hospital; later, he took me to Victoria's Secret and offered to buy me new bras and underwear (any and all that I wanted). It seemed like a great idea until we got to the store. Then all those frilly bits of lace made me cry, so we quickly left. Ben settled for giving me a teddy bear named Bergy and two lovely nightgowns that felt cool and silky smooth against my skin. He was so thoughtful, yet I had difficulty expressing my fears and weaknesses to him. I felt as if I always needed to "hang tough" even though I might want to cry.

I'd agreed to meet Ben and his parents for brunch during the Thanksgiving weekend, and I kept our date. But my reservations about being with Ben continued to grow. Even as I reassured him before and after surgery that I was going to be okay, I felt a twinge that something wasn't right with us. I think the cancer highlighted the differences between us and made me question whether he was truly the right "one" for me.

We called it quits before Christmas. Graciously, Ben still sent the bird feeder he had purchased for my family as a gift; my dad loved it. I gave my brother the gifts that I had purchased for Ben. I always enjoyed wearing the silk nightgowns he sent me, and sometimes I'm still sad that he didn't turn out to be "the one." But I knew I was right in following my instincts.

Another thing I struggled with after surgery was the fear of losing my femininity. Having breasts is so much a part of being a woman. So when I forward tips to people wanting to do something for ovarian or breast cancer survivors, I tell them, "Give or do anything that reinforces a woman's feminine feelings." Things such as manicures and pedicures, having a facial, wearing pretty silk nightgowns, picking up girly hobbies such as knitting or cross-stitching (not for me, but for others), going for a spa treatment or on a makeup-purchasing spree.

I liked massages. I liked having manicures. I liked pumicing my feet and covering my toenails with layers of polish. I liked listening to boy bands and corresponding with sorority sisters. Being a chapter advisor surrounded by young college women once a month definitely helped my healing process.

Also, I upped my subscriptions to women's magazines: *Working Woman*, *Cosmo*, *Glamour*, *Marie Claire*, *Self*, and *Shape*. I splurged on higher-thread-count sheets. I bought lots and lots of candles. I purchased or rented all the movies that Julia Roberts has starred in, and when someone sent me the first season of *Sex and the City* on DVD, I devoured it in one weekend. I put away books such as *Coaching Yourself to Success* and *How to Get Ahead in a Man's World*, and instead read *Bridget Jones's Diaries*. Both of them.

I bought a two-piece swimsuit, just to prove to myself and to others that I had two breasts, a waist, and hips. I chose clothes tailored to fit me instead of sweats and jeans. I learned to boil a three-minute egg, I baked brownies, cookies, and fruit pizzas . . . all to prove to myself that I was still a woman.

During recovery, though, being feminine was tough. For weeks after my surgery, I would wander around my townhouse like the hunchback of Notre Dame while I learned to stand up straight again. Stephanie, my housemate, was a big help. My mom, a physical therapist, showed Stephanie the least painful way to help get me out of bed while my stomach was still healing from the reconstruction surgery.

I was never hungry. Donna and Dione would come and stand over me and sing some silly made-up song about the joys of smoking pot (which I think is yucky) until I agreed to eat some chicken noodle soup just to get them to quit singing. Maybe this is not the ideal picture of postsurgery recovery: a hunchback in a silk gown, happy to have a reconstructed breast, but worried that if she didn't eat a bowl of lukewarm soup her friends would force contraband on her. But it worked for me.

Jana

As I stood in the long, winding line, waiting for the coveted front seat on the Mamba—a new super-tall, super-fast, super-scary roller coaster at the amusement park, I felt queasy. Yes, it was nearly 100 humid degrees; and yes, I was about to ride one of the tallest, fastest roller coasters in the country; but, most unsettling of all, in less than eighteen hours, my future would be determined on a surgical table.

After nearly an hour's wait, my stepmom and I climbed into the front car of the roller coaster. We were strapped in, and the ride began its slow ascent. As we crested the peak, I wondered, "What have I gotten myself into?" And then, with lightning speed, we were thrown down! Up! Down! I was in for the ride of my life. Sixty seconds later, the ride was over, and I wanted to do it again.

Looking back, I realize that my roller coaster ride was a metaphor for the next few months of my life. At the time, though, I did not realize that my life was about to become even more scary and unpredictable than the Mamba ride. And I would not want to go through those months again.

In the dark morning hours when my family and I checked in at the hospital for my lumpectomy, the roller coaster seemed a million miles away. The hospital clerk slapped an I.D. band on my wrist (name, patient number, and date of birth). The band made me feel as if now I was hospital property. In a short while, a surgical team would physically remove what remained of my cancerous lemon drop with its dirty margins, and I wouldn't know until I awoke whether or not I still had my breast; whether or not my life could be saved.

I said goodbye to my family and was taken by gurney to the operating room (OR). In the OR, the operating table seemed surprisingly narrow. Had it been so narrow in nursing school?

Lying under the surgical lights, I felt like the frog I dissected in fifth grade—completely rigid, exposed, and at the total mercy of everyone around me. Luckily, the anesthesia quickly took effect, the room blurred, and I fell asleep.

I didn't want to go through surgery twice, so I had asked my surgeon to try to spare my breast with "breast conservation surgery" (also known as a lumpectomy); but if, in her medical opinion, she was unable to obtain clean margins, she was to go ahead and remove the entire breast.

As I foggily began to "come to" after surgery, the first thing I heard was my surgeon's soft voice: "Jana, we had to remove the entire breast." I wanted to open my eyes and ask why, but I was still feeling the effects of the anesthesia. It didn't stop the wheels inside my head from spinning, though. "Why, why, why?" I wondered. Not "why" as in "Why me?" but "why" as in "What went wrong?" Why did she decide to remove my entire breast?

The pain began while I was being wheeled back to my room. Each turn of a corner made me dizzy. Once in my room, I drifted in and out of consciousness as people whispered around me. "She doesn't know." (Yes I do.) "Shhh, she needs to sleep." (I want to wake up.) "Do you think she's in pain?" (Yes, yes, yes!)

Finally, the whispering voices subsided, leaving me alone with Chris, who stayed at my side, holding my hand. When I finally opened my eyes, he told me that during surgery, my surgeon had found a second tumor. It was small—5 millimeters—and looked a lot like one of the thirteen lymph nodes she had removed, but she believed it necessitated a mastectomy. She had come out of the OR in the middle of the surgery to inform my family and get consent. My dad, as next of kin, signed the consent form. My dad, who had taught me to ride a bike, ski, throw a spiral football pass, and make stir-n-frost cake, had to give permission to remove my breast. I remember thinking these things before falling back to sleep. My dad, always there for me.

The next day, my surgeon joyfully told me that none of my lymph nodes had cancer. Such good news! Lymph node involvement helps decide the next treatment. Negative lymph node status may mean no chemotherapy. Positive status means the cancer has spread (metastasized) outside the breast to the lymph nodes, making chemotherapy likely.

As my surgeon changed my dressing and examined the mastectomy incision site, I thought, "I'm looking at the area formerly known as my breast!" From that point forward, I have always called my flat chest area just that. Sometimes I refer to my mastectomy as a "boobuscutteroffusomus" (pronounced "boob-us-cut-er-off-us-om-us"). It's so descriptive! A friend, an ovarian cancer survivor, called me the Uni-Breaster and herself, Egg Beaters.

Humor has really helped me cope with this ordeal. Early on, I decided it wouldn't do any good to take myself or my circumstances too seriously. I am always surprised when people seem offended by my lack of seriousness.

I was in the hospital for three days, and I was so grateful when my stepmom spent the night in an uncomfortable recliner that was duct-taped together just to keep me company and make sure I was okay during the night. On the second day, I saw her talking in the hallway to my dad. She had tears in her eyes, so immediately I worried. But when I asked her what was wrong, she said, "Nothing." She added, "Your dad left to run an errand. He'll be back." I fell asleep.

When I awoke, my dad was walking into my room with misty eyes. He leaned down near my bed and solemnly told me he thought I was one of the bravest people he knew, and he was proud of me. Then he reached into his pocket, pulled out one of the two Purple Heart medals he had received during his tours in Vietnam, and placed it in my hand.

When my dad was in Vietnam, he did what he had to do to serve his country, although he didn't choose to be in the situations that left him injured. Similarly, after being diagnosed with breast cancer, although I did not choose to have the disease and certainly did not want to lose a breast, I did what I had to do to save my life. I was deeply touched by Dad's gift.

Some people have told me they felt as if they were attending their own funerals when they received flowers after surgery. But

I loved every flower and the warm thoughts behind the bouquets. I felt loved, and I knew a lot of people were praying for my recovery.

I went home with two drains hanging out of my body to prevent the accumulation of fluid around the surgical site. They were safety-pinned to my shirt, and I was so afraid I would rip one of them out that I walked hunched over. Twice a day, they had to be emptied and the amount of fluid in them recorded. I hated those drains. They were cumbersome, uncomfortable, and contributed to a lot of my pain, which felt like a thousand little darts of fire shooting around the area formerly known as my breast. I was so relieved when the first drain was removed five days after surgery; a few days later, when the second drain was removed, I felt a new sense of freedom.

The first time I looked at my incision, it was scary. Without a breast, my chest appeared slightly concave with little bruising or swelling. The next scary thing was showing the "site" to Chris. He assured me he was not grossed out, and together, we measured my scar. It was nine inches long.

"I'm not marrying you for your breasts," he said. "Or breast," I corrected, causing us both to smile. But his acceptance of my new body was paramount to how I reacted to it myself. When Chris said he'd rather have me alive and healthy than with a pair of boobs and that he still thought I was beautiful, I felt immensely relieved. Feeling loved and accepted by my future mate was a major factor in maintaining a positive attitude.

Missing a breast is not easy to deal with publicly. Symmetry is important. I would be able to get a breast prosthesis (a.k.a. a fake boob) a few weeks after my incision healed, but in the meantime, I was left to my own devices. With my stepmom's help, we came up with a special arrangement of three shoulder pads from various blouses and robes she found in her closet strategically placed and pinned into my bra. As long as I didn't bounce or move too much, and with a shirt on, the shoulder pads created the illusion of a breast.

Chris was such a good sport about my shoulder-pad breast. He kept an eye on my shirt's neckline to make sure that I stayed "even." When we were out for dinner one night, he leaned over and whispered, "I see blue!" I was so caught up in the moment, I didn't know what he meant. Even when he repeated himself, I was still clueless. Finally, he told me my blue shoulder pad was peeking out of my shirt at the neckline! After a good laugh, I did some repositioning, although by now, my short-term solution was becoming a chore.

When I finally got my prescription for a breast prosthesis (no, it's not an over-the-counter item), my stepmom and I went boob shopping at the local mastectomy center. The certified "fitter" was a petite breast cancer survivor herself; she was very serious and sensitive to my needs, and she brought several styles and sizes to try on.

I was surprised there were so many choices. You can buy a fake boob with or without Velcro to adhere it to your chest. They come in various color shades so that you can closely match your skin color, and there are many sizes and shapes; and each one has a name, such as "teardrop" or "triangle." The fitting took quite a while, and in the end, I splurged on the latest edition with Velcro. I felt like a new woman. My official "breast form," made of silicone and stored in a fancy box, created the symmetry I longed for. Excitedly, I showed Chris. The touch and feel of my prosthetic breast (through a shirt, anyway) was so similar to my natural breast that he had a hard time telling which breast was real and which one was not.

Jen

Once I decided to have a mastectomy, I had just two days to wait before surgery. This was good, because it gave me very little time to think about what was going to happen. If I had watched a mastectomy being done on one of those "reality" television shows, I don't know whether I could have gone ahead with it. Even the thought of it—a surgeon making a football-shaped incision on my breast, removing the affected tissue, and then sewing together what was left—was nearly unbearable.

A big help was meeting Lisa. My church put me in touch with her because she'd been diagnosed in her early thirties. Unlike me, she wasn't pregnant at the time, but she did undergo a mastectomy and immediate reconstruction. Talking to her before surgery was very comforting. She and her two children brought me a stuffed bear with a breast cancer ribbon on its paw. I held on to that little bear before and after the surgery.

It also helped to talk to a college friend who was now a physician and knew my surgeon.

Friends and family sent e-mails and telephoned to wish me luck and calm my fears. By the morning of surgery, I was exhausted. I'd hardly slept. My mind spun with questions. What if the baby doesn't make it? What if I don't make it? Have I set everything right in my life and accomplished what God sent me here to do? What will Matt think of my new body?

When we left for the hospital, I said good-bye to our dog, Haley, as though I might not see her again. "If anything goes wrong," I told Matt, "I want them to save the baby instead of me." He grimaced and shook his head as if to say, "I don't even want to think about such an option." Filling out the hospital paperwork, which specifically outlined the risks of surgery—including death—didn't exactly help ease my fears.

My family gathered around me in pre-op, and our minister came to say a prayer. The hospital staff was monitoring the baby to check its heartbeat before surgery and they assured me that everything looked good. Still, my eyes welled with tears. I knew this was just the first hurdle in a long journey to bring a healthy baby into this world and to heal my body.

The operating room looked just as I had seen on television. Bright lights. A tray of surgical utensils. It felt cold and made me tremble. I was nervous about lying on my back for so long because at this point in pregnancy, I wasn't supposed to lie on my back anymore. The doctor marked the left side of my chest to make sure they did a mastectomy of the correct breast. The anesthesiologist put the mask over my face and I went to sleep. I started counting backwards from ten . . . the next thing I knew I was waking up in the recovery room.

The procedure took about an hour, though it felt like an eternity to my family. My surgeon told me that everything had gone beautifully and the baby and I were doing great. To my family, he explained that although he didn't see anything in my lymph nodes, we would have to wait for the final pathology report to know for sure.

My hospital room was small, so my family came in shifts; Matt first. Flowers arrived in droves. I even received flowers from the Zeta chapter of my college sorority. Matt and I were serving on the Baker University alumni board at that time, and the director was also the Zeta chapter adviser. I thought it was incredibly sweet of the House to think of me when none of them really knew who I was.

I slept a lot the first day, holding on tightly to the little bear Lisa had given me. I wanted to lie on my left side because that's the best side to lie on when pregnant, but I hurt too much.

By evening, I was hungry, and ate just about everything on my plate. To my embarrassment—especially since my family was there—it all came back up. Obviously, the effects of anesthesia were still with me. After that, I was restricted to liquids until the next morning.

Like the good mother she is, my mom stayed overnight with me, but between nurses coming in to check my vitals and my roommate clearing her throat every five minutes (she had undergone thyroid surgery), neither of us got much sleep.

Matt and my mom were with me when the surgeon removed the bandages from my chest. I knew I had lost my breast, but I was not prepared to see the awful-looking scar that went from my sternum into my armpit. I was as flat as a pancake, even slightly concave. I felt like a seven-year-old again, only without a nipple.

The surgeon asked whether I was okay. I took a deep breath and glanced at Matt. He hadn't flinched, which is one of the greatest gifts he ever gave to me.

When it was time to leave the hospital, I didn't want people to know I had lost my breast. I put on my bra, which hurt, and stuffed the left side with socks. Thank goodness my pregnant belly distracted attention from my chest. Still, I hoped no one could tell.

At home, my mom stayed with me for two days while Matt finished the school semester. While there, she put up our Christmas tree. I lay on the couch and helped a little, but my heart wasn't in it. I kept thinking, "What if this is my last Christmas?"

Besides teaching, Matt helped coach basketball, and his team had its first game two days after my surgery. I had never missed one of his games, and I wasn't about to start. Since I couldn't lift my left arm because of the lymph node dissection, my mom helped me bathe. She was afraid I was pushing myself and tried to convince me not to go to the game, but I insisted. When we headed to the school gym, I had socks stuffed in my bra and the drains were tucked under my shirt.

As I sat in the stands, Matt's head coach saw me. I could tell he thought I looked awful. I think my presence at the game surprised a lot of people. It might even have made them uncomfortable. One of Matt's basketball players had battled leukemia the year before and he said hello. It inspired me to realize that he looked healthy and was able to play basketball again. In hindsight, though, my mom was right. I probably should have skipped the game.

After losing my breast, all I seemed to see on television were scantily clad women flaunting their voluptuous breasts. I felt as though I was the only young woman in the world who had ever lost a breast. Even the American Cancer Society booklet showed older women modeling breast forms and wigs. I kept asking Matt whether he was okay with my new body image. He always reassured me: "You're more beautiful than ever."

A friend of my aunt's had a niece who had been diagnosed while pregnant, and it helped to talk to her. She was diagnosed very late in her pregnancy, so she didn't undergo chemotherapy while pregnant, but she did have surgery. It was such a relief to hear that her son was born healthy. She had just had her second child, which further encouraged me because Matt and I had always wanted two children—a boy and then, we hoped, a girl.

When my surgeon called to tell me that there was no cancer in the nineteen lymph nodes he'd removed, I started jumping up and down in delight. My chances for long-term survival had just increased dramatically. And I would need only four rounds of chemotherapy. My final diagnosis was Stage IIa, invasive ductal carcinoma.

Within a few days, the liquid flowing into the drains had slowed considerably and I was able to have them removed. It hurt when the surgeon removed them, but I left his office a liberated woman. Now I just needed something other than a sock for my bra!

My surgeon put me in touch with a woman who could fit me for a postsurgery bra. She came to my house, which made the process more tolerable. Only the surgeon, my mom, and Matt had seen my chest since the surgery, and I was worried about letting other people see it. I didn't know you're not supposed to wear a bra after surgery while your body is healing. The woman gave me a camisole that had a pocket on the left side in which I could place cotton filling. It was lightweight and made me feel more comfortable. Now I could go back into the office and not feel like a freak.

Originally, Matt and I had wanted our baby's sex to be a surprise, but before I started chemotherapy, we changed our minds. With everything going on in our lives, we wanted some certainty. Matt was convinced we were having a little girl, but as the technician looked at the sonogram, she quickly pronounced, "It's a boy!" My mom was there and kept asking, "But how can you tell?"—which made the rest of us smile.

My chest was healing nicely; there were no complications from the surgery. I was scheduled to start chemotherapy two weeks after surgery. I asked again whether we might delay it for the baby's sake, but my doctor said we had to take care of it. The time had come to do battle against any remaining cancer cells in my body!

Kim

So, my choice was made. I would have a mastectomy with a TRAM flap reconstruction. I had never had surgery before, so I was scared. To take my mind off what was coming, my wonderful husband rented a hotel suite the weekend before my surgery, and we pretended we were on vacation. We went out to dinner, rented movies, drank wine, and had great sex. It was a perfect weekend. Our last weekend before my body changed forever.

The day before surgery, my best friends took me to lunch, and my friend Laura took me shopping for nightgowns. "If you're going to be in the hospital, you want to look presentable," she said. Maybe not a glamorous negligee, but at least a nice gown. We had a great time shopping, but as I browsed the sleepwear section, I kept thinking about losing a breast and how I might never look the same. It really hit me in the face as I stood in the dressing room and tried on "comfy" old-woman gowns instead of sexy nighties.

Brandon was staying with Scott's parents while I was in the hospital. For him it was a treat, but as I put him in his grandparents' car, tears rolled down my face. I kept thinking about the "what if's." What if something goes wrong?

I also had fears about losing a part of me. Would my husband look at me the same way? Would I ever regain feeling in my new reconstructed breast? Would I be able to breast-feed if we decided to have more children? Would I be able to wear a bathing suit? Would I feel like a complete woman?

I knew my breast was a dispensable part of my body. I didn't need it to survive. But I felt an attachment to my right breast. It had been good to me through the years—giving my husband much joy and feeding my son for the first few months of his life. I felt I should have some sort of memorial service as I said good-bye to something that had been a part of me for thirty-one years.

Mostly, though, I feared that if something went wrong and I didn't make it, Brandon would be too little to remember his mommy. I took a lot of pictures right before surgery. I even thought about making him a video, but Scott wouldn't let me do that. Instead, I wrote him a letter. I also prepared a living will and a power of attorney. I wanted to be prepared for the "just in case."

As my fears played out in my mind the night before surgery, Scott's mom asked us to join her in a prayer. I have always been a spiritual person, although Scott and I did not belong to a church. However, at that moment, standing with my hands held by Scott and his mom, I felt more in touch with God than I ever had. I begged Him to save me so I could be a mommy and a wife to the two most important people in my life.

Unlike the other Nordie Girls, I had gone through chemotherapy before surgery, so my veins were shot. After trying several times and failing to get an IV in, the nurses decided to put in the IV after I had been knocked out, which was fine by me. I just wondered why they hadn't decided that before they made me a human pin cushion. As they wheeled me off for surgery, I took one last look at my breast; I realized that in a matter of hours it would be gone forever.

The surgery began at 7:30 A.M. and lasted about six hours. My breast surgeon performed the mastectomy and lymph node dissection in a little over an hour. Then the plastic surgeon took over to begin the reconstruction. Because the arteries in my chest were not supplying enough blood to keep the new tissue alive, she changed her procedure. Instead of completely removing the abdominal tissue and reattaching it in my chest (free flap reconstruction), she opted to keep the arteries intact and tunnel the tissue up to my chest (pedicel flap reconstruction). It was nothing unusual, just a different means to the same end.

Here's one way to picture the procedure. My breast surgeon cut open my right breast and hollowed it out like a pumpkin, removing all my breast tissue and a mass of lymph nodes. Then, my plastic surgeon and her team took my abdominal tissue, muscles, and skin, tunneled it up through my abdomen, and used it to build my new breast. They even moved my belly button to make everything symmetrical.

When I woke up after surgery and Scott told me they had done the procedure differently, I asked only one question: "Did they still take my fat and give me a tummy tuck?" My family and friends in the room laughed.

For the first three days in the hospital, I used a personal pain pump, and morphine became my friend. My abdominal area was excruciatingly painful.

I got out of bed for the first time on my second day after surgery. It hurt to move, but I managed to make it to the recliner. My appetite came back on the third day, and hospital food tasted much better this time than it did after I gave birth to Brandon. I had my own room, and when I wanted to eat, I called down and ordered whatever I wanted off the menu. It was like room service.

The visitors, cards, phone calls, and flowers were the best gifts I could have received after my surgery. Every day, Scott read me the cards and comments from the Web site we had created to update family and friends. It was the love from family and friends that kept me going while I was in the hospital.

Like the other Nordie Girls, I could hardly wait to have the drains in my abdomen and chest removed. I was less eager to say goodbye to my pain pump, which they took away on the third day. I was then switched to oral medications. That same day, my breast surgeon informed us that the fifteen lymph nodes she had removed had no involvement. Scott and I were so excited!

This was also the day I decided to look at my new breast for the first time. I asked Scott to bring me a mirror. Anxiously, I removed the bandages. There was my new breast, made out of my stomach tissue. Although a bit discolored, it looked like a real breast (minus the nipple and areola, which would be put on later). However, it didn't feel like a breast. It was completely numb. The doctors had told me to expect this. Eventually, I might get partial feeling back, they explained.

When they told me I could go home, five days after surgery, I was scared. Just getting up to go to the bathroom was a chore, and I couldn't do it alone. Scott had to help me take a shower. How would I manage at home?

The good news was that I would go home without my drains. My surgeon said she didn't think she had ever before sent anyone home without the drains. I was an overachiever, even as a cancer patient!

At home, I slept most of the time for the next two weeks. My mom brought Brandon to visit three weeks after surgery. I still couldn't hold him, but it was wonderful to see him. I had missed him so much.

Gradually, I gained strength. I followed the doctor's orders and diligently did the physical therapy exercises for my arm so that I wouldn't lose arm mobility. It took me seven weeks to walk without looking like the hunchback of Notre Dame. Scott called me "Mr. Burns" from the television show *The Simpsons* because I walked hunched over, dragging my right arm.

Scott was wonderful during this time. I've always been so independent. It was humbling to need my husband to give me a bath and get me dressed. That's when you know you have found true love.

Several times the stitches in my stomach opened up, and my doctors lectured me: "Kim, you have to slow down. You're doing too much." I tried to listen. I sat in a recliner more than I care to for the rest of my life.

I took six weeks off from work. After that, I was at least able to use a laptop and work from home. At times, I felt I was losing my sanity. I wanted to be the old me, bouncing around from event to event. Scott would remind me, "Kim, you just had half of your body cut open." When he put it that way, I knew he was right. My surgery taught me to listen to my body and rest when I felt tired. It was a huge lesson for me.

Recovering from surgery was, in some ways, worse than chemotherapy. I couldn't ignore my physical exhaustion. I couldn't pick up my son. And Brandon had to stay with his grandparents for six weeks, which was a long time when he couldn't understand what was happening.

While I recuperated, we switched Brandon to his big-boy bed (a fire truck) and had him start eating at his big-boy table instead of in his high chair. Although it worked out well, I felt as though I'd taken away part of his childhood and forced him to grow up too fast.

It was a long time before I slept well at night. I was proud of my new flat tummy, though. I could get into my pre-pregnancy clothes! But even with a shirt on, you could definitely tell I had two different boobs—one was hanging about a foot lower than the other. My new breast was perky; the old one sagged. It's amazing what motherhood can do to your breasts. Because of the pain, I decided to switch to button-down shirts. It would have been better if I had known this before surgery instead of trying to shop for them while recuperating.

During those first few weeks at home, I often stood and looked at myself in the mirror. My new breast looked like a breast, but it didn't have much sensation. Would Scott and I still have great sex? Would I get as aroused without sensation in my breast? And yes, I wondered how I would look in a swimsuit. I was definitely not wearing sexy bras. In fact, I didn't wear a bra at all for six weeks. When I did start, I could no longer wear underwire bras because they irritated my scar. Try finding sexy bras with no underwire—not easy.

The scar that ran across my abdomen from hip bone to hip bone was also very noticeable. I called it my "smiley face" and used Mederma to help it lighten in time—and it did. I thought of my scars as battle scars—a battle that I had won. Although I didn't look like the supermodels on the covers of *Vogue* or *Cosmo*, I was comfortable with the new me.

But would Scott be? The answer came the first time we had sex after my surgery. He just kept telling me how beautiful I was and that he loved me for me. Now I know why I married this man.

I never wanted to be judged solely on my boobs or my body. But we live in such a breast-obsessed society. Breasts are everywhere—in magazines, on billboards, on television. After my surgery, boobs seemed to be a constant presence. One day, I caught myself looking in a mirror and feeling sorry for myself. Wham! It hit me. I was not going to let myself become a victim. The pity-party was over. I just had to accept my new body, remember that beauty truly does come from within, and realize that I was still the same person.

Once I recovered from my TRAM flap reconstruction, I had my nipple reconstructed and my unaffected breast lifted. Fortunately, insurance covered the breast lift, so my "mommy" boob, as I call it (thanks to breast-feeding) didn't sag any more. However, I had to wait six months for these surgeries because, although I had no lymph node involvement, we had decided to do another four rounds of chemotherapy because of my age and the aggressive nature of my cancer.

My plastic surgeon did my nipple reconstruction and breast lift at the same time. By this time, I was an old pro at surgeries. This would be my fourth in less than a year. The nipple reconstruction and breast lift were outpatient procedures and fairly simple, although I experienced more pain with the breast lift than I had expected. Once again, painkillers became my friend.

Unfortunately, the nipple reconstruction required a second procedure, but eventually it turned out well. The new nipple is a little smaller and doesn't get hard like my real one, but it is a nipple. The last procedure was my areola tattoo, but I needed laser hair removal first because hair started growing on my breast as though the skin were still on my abdomen. Patti suggested that I do the laser hair removal before my tattoo; this was something she wished she had done differently. Once again, Patti's support was invaluable. I'm not actually sure I'll ever get the areola tattoo—maybe I'll get a pink ribbon tattoo on my breast instead. Who needs an areola, anyway?

Cancer surgery made me laugh at myself more. I also lost any modesty I ever had concerning my body. Patti helped ease my fears by showing me her reconstruction. I vowed to do the same, and now I will pull up my shirt for breast cancer patients to show them my TRAM flap reconstruction. It took a while, but now I accept the new me.

CHAPTER FIVE

Chemotherapy: Bald Is Beautiful

— Nordie's Café —
October 2002

ctober is National Breast Cancer Awareness Month. Every one of us had become activists, willing to go public in order to encourage awareness and research. It meant a month of clipboards and checklists, too many voicemails and computer voices telling us "you have . . . three hundred new e-mails." Each morning we put on nice attire, coifed our hair, and made our faces ready for television, even though at times we secretly wanted a break from our nonstop schedules.

Our monthly luncheon started out with a bit of venting—but by our third bite we were talking about the opportunity the month afforded us to educate others about breast cancer. This energy moved us along.

Our discussion shifted to the book and our next chapter: chemotherapy. Jana asked, "What do women need to know about going through chemo? What did we need to know? Sure, there's hair loss—and the medical stuff I like to talk about—but what is chemo really like?"

"It starts with the Kool-Aid color chemo mixes. 'I'll have one with one part red, one part clear, in a bag—and I'll take care of the needle,'" said Patti, mimicking a bar order. "But it's not like Kool-Aid because it makes you feel like shit."

"There's the hair loss and the wig problem," murmured Jen, thinking out loud.

"Yeah, it's pretty ridiculous the way women try to hold onto some small clump of hair," said Kim. "On the plus side, no shaving for several months," offered Jen. "And you save money on hair products, hair cuts, and highlights."

"And it sure shortens the getting-ready time in the morning," added Jana, laughing. "Doesn't take much time to pop on a hat or wig!"

We ended lunch by going back to our calendars. October was a full month, and Kim happened to be going through it bald. It gave her hope to see Jana, Jen, and Patti—proof positive that her hair would grow back. In the meantime, we agreed that on our next meeting date each of us would have written our memories of chemo—and how each of us discovered that bald really can be beautiful.

Patti

For me, one of the toughest parts of having cancer was losing my hair. It came out first little by little, then in clumps. No matter how little or softly I brushed it, it kept falling out.

I began chemotherapy after surgery, even though the lab hadn't found any cancer in my lymph tissue. My oncologist suggested the treatments "just to be sure." I had four treatments of Adriamycin and Cytoxan administered at three-week intervals for three months. I opted out of Tamoxifen because it probably wouldn't decrease my chance of recurrence; besides, I've never been a fan of taking unnecessary pills.

I decided to have my treatments on Friday afternoons so that my work week wouldn't be interrupted. Donna accompanied me, and other friends usually stopped by during the three-hour infusion. One way I passed time was answering love quizzes from *Cosmopolitan* with the older women getting treatment! I ended the day at home eating pizza and playing cards with friends. Then I hibernated for the weekend—the start of my three-week chemo cycle.

The first week I didn't feel nauseous, just a bit sluggish.

The second week was hard. My blood counts hit their lowest and my exhaustion was greatest. One Friday, my blood counts were exceptionally low—only thirty-six white blood cells per deciliter; most chemo patients have a thousand, and the normal number is ten thousand. My doctor talked about hospitalizing me, but I told her that was "out of the question."

After that round with my oncologist, I went home and became the "bubble girl" for the weekend. My housemate, Stephanie, and I disinfected my entire condo so that I could stay healthy as long as I stayed inside. Even a cold would have hospitalized me. During most second weeks, I just tried to keep my head above water.

The third week, my energy peaked, so that was when I scheduled everything: baby showers, working lunches, bar nights. For that week, I was a woman about town.

Hair loss affected me on two levels: comfort and appearance. Hair keeps your head comfortably warm. I was getting my treatments in the winter. Brrrrrr. A friend gave me a fabulous hat, lined with silky material that felt great against my sensitive bald head. (Chemo dries you out all over, and your head, especially, can become tender and itchy.)

I loved this hat because it was a leopard print; it fairly screamed, "Look at me, I have no hair, but I'm not afraid to go out, have fun, and be outrageously proud of the fact that I'm still here!" I wore it when I needed a self-confidence boost, or when I just wanted to have fun.

My other favorite thing for keeping my head warm was an old worn-out red bandana that I wore around the house and in bed at night. I used Sap Moss shampoo and conditioner from Aveda to keep my scalp and any hair that was left moisturized.

More than the appearance of baldness, I hated the stares and questions.

I bought a wig that was itchy and didn't look like any haircut I'd ever had. But I wore it whenever I wanted anonymity—when I went shopping at the mall for Christmas presents or when I attended a basketball game.

One night for a formal business party, I "glammed out" with a blonde wig. I felt like Gwyneth Paltrow and made sure I was photographed to commemorate my "night as a blonde." However, when I went back to work on Monday, I was happy to leave the blonde wig at home.

Along with my hair, my eyebrows fell out. Eyebrows are more important than you might think, and facial expressions are hard to master when they're not there. I wish I had visited a couple of makeup counters and practiced with brow pencils to get the shaping right *before* my hair started to fall out.

Besides baldness, I experienced a lot of bloody noses from chemo. At work, I'd sit at the customer help desk, my head-set on, Kleenex stuffed up my nose, head back, feet propped up—all the while explaining to customers the ins and outs of their computer problems.

When my nose finally did stop bleeding, it was raw and sore, so I carried around saline spray, Puffs tissues, and Vaseline—surely one of life's greatest inventions. I've yet to find anything better for soothing cracked lips, raw noses, and diarrhea bottom.

For mouth sores—another chemo side effect—I ate a lot of yogurt and popsicles, and added Dutch-chocolate-flavored Ensure for protein. In the first two weeks of the three-week cycle, I couldn't taste anything, so I concentrated on texture foods, such as broccoli and granola bars. I ate so much broccoli that I'm surprised I don't hate it, but it's still one of my favorite foods.

During week three, when my appetite came back, I gorged myself on as many spicy and aromatic foods as I could stomach.

Since cancer was not in my lymph nodes, once I had made it through the three months of precautionary chemo, I could put the entire experience behind me. That knowledge kept me going, and even allowed me to have some fun. I sent clumps of hair to my brother in Africa as a Christmas present and wrote this note:

My hair continues to grow back thick and curly, but darker than before. Had a brief health scare at my six-month check-up when my surgeon had me do a mammogram for some lumpy areas in my right breast—but all tests came back OK. It was nightmarish though, and I'm looking into a couple of visits with a psychologist to get some "tools" for dealing with the rest of my life.

Logically, there's almost no way I should get cancer again. After the surgery, I had a bone scan that showed the cancer did *not* get into my bones, *nor* did the cancer make it to my lymph nodes. Therefore, it did *not* spread past the breast tissue. The three months of chemo were just to make sure there was no cancer left. All my postchemo tests came back great. But logic has little pull when your surgeon asks you to get a second mammogram "as a precaution."

When my hair started growing back, I confidently scheduled an appointment with my hairstylist, Tracy. After months of trying to "fake it," he sounded genuinely excited about having a real head of hair to work on rather than a scalp of clumpy locks to "manage," or simply a bald head to massage. In college and beyond, my hair was lighter than now, so I planned to have highlights put in; but when I saw the look on Tracy's face, I anticipated his first words: "Not a lot to highlight here." He was kind, though. He was happy my hair was coming back and with it our lively visits. So was I.

In retrospect, it seems as if I almost "played" at having cancer. I literally laid out a timeline with goals and objectives, and then marched forward to achieve them. I cried only twice, both times with Donna. The first time I lost control was the day before my first chemo treatment. Sitting alone in my apartment, I suddenly felt so lonely. The second time it happened, I was heading home for Christmas and I realized that, physically, I was not the person I'd been a year ago. Both times, all Donna could do was let me blubber and rock back and forth as I wept about not having the "body that was given to me."

Since then, I've learned not only to love my new body, but to appreciate it fully. My abdomen will be eternally flat. I got the insurance-paid breast reduction that I had always wanted, and my hair grew back. I'd say I have better body confidence now than I ever had. I count it as one of my daily blessings.

Jana

Giant tears rolled down my cheeks as my stepmom drove me to my first chemotherapy appointment. I'm not sure what made me cry. Maybe sheer terror at the chemotherapy horror stories I'd heard. Stories about relentless vomiting, hair loss, fainting, and other bad reactions. Maybe it was fear of the unknown. What if the treatments didn't work? I was prepared to do whatever I had to do to save my life. I was not prepared to go through a mastectomy and chemotherapy with no results.

Even though my lymph node sites were clear and my cancer was at Stage I, like Patti, I opted for chemotherapy as a preventive measure—"just in case." Several factors influenced my decision. First, my cancer was "multifocal"—a second tumor had been discovered during surgery. Also, I was unusually young, and the genesis of my breast cancer was unknown. I was healthy enough physically to tolerate the toxic treatments. And finally, my oncologist advised chemotherapy.

I would receive four cycles of two drugs, Adriamycin and Cytoxan. If things went according to my math, counting the three weeks between treatment cycles, I would finish my fourth and final treatment one month before my wedding. Whew! I could get married as scheduled.

But I wasn't thinking about getting married as I nervously waited with my stepmom for my first treatment. My fellow waiting-roomers, I noticed, were all older people, most of them in their golden years. Even their children, who accompanied some of them, were my parents' ages! I noticed a sign in the room. Ironically, it said "No Children."

Others in the thirty-seat waiting room seemed to look at me with shock and sadness when I made eye contact. In hindsight, this was probably half fact and half my own self-consciousness.

In the treatment room, twenty La-Z-Boy-type vinyl recliners circled the nurses' station. Curtain dividers could be pulled for privacy, although in such a small room, there was no privacy. I selected my recliner—my home—for the next three hours. A nurse told my stepmom that she could sit in the recliner next to mine, though she'd have to give it up if a patient needed it. For future infusions, she brought her own pop-up chair and sat beside me.

Patients in the other recliners wore baseball hats, turbans, wigs, or nothing at all; most had obviously lost their hair. Each patient seemed to be in his or her own little world. Some curled up under fleece blankets. Some chatted with visitors. Some ate fast food. Some slept; one was even snoring loudly. The chemotherapy clinic had a palpable "feeling." A feeling of hope, despair, fear, and sadness. And one common denominator: Human life is fragile, but humans are strong and life is worth fighting for.

My treatment officially began when the saline solution dripped into my IV, and was soon supplemented by several "piggy back" bags of fluid (as soon as one bag finished, the next would start, until all were empty. Then the saline would drip again). Some patients, whose medications required precise timing and delivery, were hooked up to fancy electronic IV pumps, but mine were based on a low-tech concept: gravity.

In addition to the saline, I received a bag of Decadron, a bag of Zofran, and a bag of Cytoxan. As I looked around the room, I momentarily felt important because I had so many bags: four. A neighboring patient only had two. Oh, wait, a patient across from me had five or six. I guess I wasn't so important after all. (Even in treatment I could be competitive!)

I took two drugs in addition to the four drip bags. They were inserted into my vein through a portal on the IV tubing. Ativan required a small syringe and only a few seconds to administer. Adriamycin, which looked like cherry Kool-Aid, was administered through a jumbo-sized syringe, and had to be given very carefully. If it infiltrated through a vein into my tissue, it could cause necrosis, or tissue death. That was a pretty unnerving thought.

When we headed home, I felt "woozy," but not too bad, though I made sure to overlap my cocktail of anti-nausea drugs—a mixture of Ativan, Compazine, and Decadron. I took them faithfully every five hours—even in the middle of the night—and though I felt nauseous and became constipated, the cocktail kept me from vomiting. The drugs also caused drowsiness, but hey, I didn't mind sleeping through it all!

At one point during my chemotherapy, I had an epiphany of sorts, when one day, as I gazed out my bedroom window and watched the traffic going past, I realized the world was still going—without me! That's when I decided I needed to make a difference in this world. I would find a way to make a positive impact with my life so the world would at least notice if I was not in it.

My chemotherapy treatments targeted and killed not only cancer cells but healthy cells, too. Six days into my first chemotherapy, when all my cells were at their lowest point from the toxic drugs (called my "nadir"), I lay on the couch and moaned to my dad, "I feel horrible."

"Jana, of course you do," he exclaimed, "the chemotherapy is killing you!" I had never looked at it quite that way before. If I was to live, good cells as well as the bad ones must die. Yes. No wonder I felt so bad. Four days later, my hair began to fall out as I brushed my bangs. Oh, shit. It's happening. It's really happening. I thought I was prepared. I'd cut my shoulder-length hair very short, and I'd gone wig shopping with my sister. We had bought a "fun wig" that was short and dark brown, and another wig that matched my real hair style and color almost exactly. I called it my "wedding wig." But it was still traumatic when the first strands of hair fell out.

At first, I planned to let nature take its course. But there's nothing natural about losing your hair! I got impatient. In a perverse sort of way, it intrigued me to tug gently on a tuft of hair and see it come out. I decided I'd rather pull it out than have it show up on my pillow or in the shower drain. So I pulled out all except for a strip along the middle of my head. I had a Mohawk! I sprayed my Mohawk into place and went downstairs to show my dad.

After his initial shock, he suggested that I go to the mall to see whether the punk-rocker teenagers would think I was cool. "I do not find that amusing," I countered.

Later that same evening, after showing off my Mohawk to Chris, I asked him to help pull out the rest of my hair. What a strange date! When all my hair was gone, I inspected my head. No strange purple birthmark. No funny bumps or lumps. In fact, I had a pretty fine-looking head. Chris kissed my bald head and told me I was pretty, with or without hair. His love and support helped me accept my baldness.

One final thing about hair loss: Yes, Virginia, every single hair on your body does fall out. Even eyelashes and eyebrows. Wearing false eyelashes and fake eyebrows to my wedding was unthinkable, so my girlfriends started a separate prayer chain to supplement the prayer chain about my health in general. They prayed that I would not lose all of my eyebrows and eyelashes. Their prayers were answered. Although my brows and lashes thinned, I did not lose them all.

I had asked my oncologist whether I would gain or lose weight during chemotherapy, and she told me that neither would happen. She was correct. For about a week, my appetite disappeared, but then it became normal again. Except for food cravings. One craving I had was for cherry-chip cookies (found only in Colorado). Fortunately, my friend Heidi express-mailed a dozen to me, and I happily ate them all in one day. A less difficult craving to satisfy was my desire for Rice Krispies topped with banana slices. Nothing else would do. So despite my fatigue, I drove to the grocery store to buy the food. "Why am I doing this?" I wondered as I pushed my cart around the produce section.

That's when I ran into the mango display. Literally. My cart knocked over the entire display, spilling mangos everywhere. As I bent down to pick then up, I nearly fainted. Visions of passing out and having someone call 911 ran through my head. Through sheer will and the fear of 911, I mustered enough energy to find a grocery store employee to help pick up the mangos. I escaped the store with neither bananas nor Rice Krispies. For ten minutes, I just sat in my car and tried to gather enough strength to drive home.

I had a hard time letting people do things for me, although I really enjoyed and appreciated it when they did. One day, I e-mailed a coworker, Christine, and asked whether she could drop off some instant cocoa mix on her way home because I was craving hot chocolate. She didn't know what type of cocoa I liked, so she bought me every flavor Swiss Miss makes. I had no idea there were so many cocoa options! It was great.

Another friend, Rochelle, bought me my two favorite hats (as Patti said, a bald head gets extremely cold—especially at night). I called one my "thinking cap" because on the front it had a little smiling guy and the phrase "Life is Good." (I have since discovered that his name is Jake—visit www.lifeisgood.com.) This phrase became one of my mantras. I even bought a fund-raising brick for a renovation project that had "Life is good!" engraved on it.

The other hat was a sort of surgeon's cap with pictures of hens and eggs on it. It fit snugly and kept my head warm each night. I called it my "chicken cap."

For fun, Jill, a cancer survivor, loaned me her *Flashdance* wig. It looked like Jennifer Beals's frizzy big brown hair in the 1980s movie. I put on the wig and greeted my future in-laws at the door. "Do you like my new hairstyle?" I asked. It took a couple of minutes for them to realize I was joking. Then we all had a good laugh.

By week number three, as my cells reproduced and replaced the cells killed by the chemo, I felt better. I had enough energy to captain my own team in the Komen Race for the Cure, which was being held that week. Family, friends, and coworkers came out in force to participate on "Team JKL" (my initials). To my surprise and delight, I was honored as the captain of that year's largest community team.

The Race for the Cure was almost awe-inspiring for me. I was completely overwhelmed to see hundreds of breast cancer survivors in hot pink tee shirts and to realize that I was among them. It was my first weekend with my wig (yes, I was so vain that I wore my wig!), and I was one of the last to cross the finish line in the one-mile fun walk. All my weaknesses were apparent. The experience was surreal, and left me feeling strangely alone. Even though I was among a crowd of people—including family and friends who were there to support me that day—I did not fit in with the other pink-tee-shirt-wearing breast cancer survivors. In spite of having lost a breast to my mastectomy, having lost my hair to chemotherapy, and having cried a lifetime's worth of tears, I had never let it truly sink in that I had breast cancer. I was only twenty-seven years old.

Treatment number two was eventful only because I had mouth sores during my nadir. Long cuts extended along my gum lines, and my whole mouth hurt. The clinic nurses gave me a prescription for something called "velvet glove." It not only numbed my gums but also my entire mouth and tongue, and it was almost worse than the mouth sores. When I learned that they were "going to get worse," I cried the whole way home. Fortunately, my friend Jill told me about an over-the-counter mouthwash she had used called Biotene. I used it faithfully and my mouth sores lessened.

Because treatments one and two had been relatively uneventful, other than the mango and mouth-sore incidents, I thought treatment number three would be a breeze. It was not. I got a bad cold and lost all my white blood cells. I was forced to take infection-control prevention measures, which meant, among other things, not eating any fresh fruits or veggies (of course, I was craving strawberries and baby carrots . . . sigh). When I was told to wear a mask in public places such as malls or movie theaters, I just stayed home. My muscles ached so severely I could barely move. I was wiped out.

The day after treatment number four—the last round before my wedding—something new occurred. The big toe on
my left foot suddenly turned bright red. In addition, it was excruciatingly painful. On a scale of 1 to 10, with 10 being the
worst, my pain was a 12. By the next morning, my other toes
and fingertips were flame red and painful, and as I left for the
doctor's office, I began to get tiny red spots on my hands. I
started to panic. What was going on?

No one seemed to know. My oncologist was out that week,
and the covering doctor thought it might be gout. For an entire
day, I treated my now worsening symptoms with gout medication. No improvement. My primary care physician was perplexed and referred me to a dermatologist. The dermatologist
was also perplexed, and after consulting his partner, he decided
to biopsy one of the lesions. Meanwhile, I could barely walk
because the pain was so bad. The dermatologist referred me to
a cardiologist, "just in case it's bacterial endocarditis." Great.
Now I have to worry about my heart? The cardiologist wanted
to do a transesophageal echocardiogram (TEE). In this procedure, a tube with a fiber optic camera on the end is put down
the esophagus so the doctor can view the heart valves from the
inside. If he saw bacterial endocarditis, I would be admitted to
the hospital immediately for long-term antibiotic treatment.

The night before my TEE procedure, I lay in bed in intense
and unrelenting pain. I felt the pain not just at the spots of
redness and swelling on my fingers and toes; it was now shooting sharply up and down my hands, arms, legs, and feet. All
night, I prayed and prayed and prayed. I was afraid I was dying.
I was afraid I would not get married. I remember thinking that
my pain was only a fraction of what Jesus must have endured
when He was crucified, and this gave me strength. That night

is forever imprinted in my memory. After I made it through that, I believed I could make it through anything.

The TEE was negative, which was both good and bad news. Good because I did not have bacterial endocarditis. Bad because I was still labeled "diagnosis unknown," and my symptoms worsened each day. The cardiologist recommended that I see an immunologist, but before I saw the immunologist, I had my blood drawn for the fifth time that week to rule out a systemic infection. After twenty-four and forty-eight hours, the blood tests were negative. Again, that was good and bad news.

Meanwhile, my dermatologist's office lost the biopsy specimen, so there were no pathology results from my lesions. By the time I saw the immunologist, the eighth specialist I had seen in five days, I was so weak that my dad drove me to our appointment.

The immunologist thought I was having a toxic reaction to chemotherapy and was experiencing an autoimmune response called "vasculitis." Although he couldn't confirm this diagnosis until his own bloodwork tests came back, he gave me a shot of a corticosteroid and a prescription for Prednisone, an oral corticosteroid. Within hours, my pain began to subside. The corticosteroids are wonder drugs for stopping the inflammatory process.

Blood tests confirmed the immunologist's diagnosis of vasculitis, and he continued to treat me, even after my final chemotherapy treatment. The vasculitis caused my toenails and fingernails on the affected fingers to fall off, so my sister had to glue on false nails for my wedding.

Chemotherapy left me with a new feeling of vulnerability. It forced me to slow down, and helped me appreciate small highlights during my day, such as going to the mailbox to see who had sent RSVPs to our wedding invitations.

I also had time to read, a pastime I'd enjoyed in childhood. I devoured everything in print, starting with the breast cancer bible: *Dr. Susan Love's Breast Book*. From there I read medical textbooks that I checked out from a local medical school library. Once I was satisfied I knew everything I could about breast cancer, I switched gears and read inspirational, then humorous books. Moving on to nonfiction and fiction, I read it all. Once again, I was a bookworm.

Finally, after four rounds of chemotherapy, losing my hair and fingernails, and surviving vasculitis, it was time for me to get married!

I walked down the aisle with my fake boob sewn into my gown, and with my wedding wig on my head. I married Chris— as scheduled! Dreams of our wedding and our future together helped me stay focused on getting through the tough times. And my faith in God gave me strength when I needed it most.

Jen

Before beginning chemotherapy, I underwent a multigated acquisition (MUGA) scan, a procedure that evaluates the pumping function of the heart ventricles. This was necessary because one of the drugs I needed, Adriamycin, can be toxic to the heart. The technician hooked me up to a machine on my left side, the same side as the mastectomy. I started crying, embarrassed that yet another person would see my disfigured body. Poor guy. He tried to keep things light with small talk, but I was in no mood to respond.

My mom went with me to my first chemo treatment. I was terrified! The infusion room was full of recliners and people hooked up to IVs, and, as Jana said, the average age was easily sixty. I looked at all these older people with scarves, hats, and wigs hiding their bald heads, and I felt as if I were having an out-of-body experience. I couldn't believe I was being treated for cancer. As I read the paperwork I had to sign, and noted all the complications that could occur during chemotherapy, I felt as if I were signing my life away.

The nurses assured me that the molecules in the chemotherapy I was taking were large enough not to pass through the placenta and harm my baby, but I was still scared. When they hooked me up to the IV, my eyes filled with tears. What was this doing to our child? I prayed to God to keep our son safe and asked Him for some sort of sign.

Adriamycin's bright red color surprised me. No wonder it's nicknamed "the red devil." It was administered through an IV in my hand, and it felt so ice cold going into my veins that I began to shiver.

I had gotten used to going to the bathroom every half hour during pregnancy. So, in the middle of treatment, I wheeled my IV into the restroom. I was frantic when I saw the color red in the toilet bowl. Was something wrong with our baby? Was I miscarrying? I flew out of the restroom to tell the nurses. They had forgotten to tell me that Adriamycin turns urine red temporarily. What a relief. But I still felt a little spooked that it had gone through my system so quickly.

My treatments occurred every third Wednesday, so I worked from home the following Thursday and Friday. The doctors had wanted me to take medical leave, but I didn't want too much time to think about the seriousness of my situation. And I wanted to take a full twelve weeks off when our baby was born.

On Wednesdays between treatments, I had my blood levels checked. If I didn't have enough infection-fighting white blood cells, a minor infection could become life threatening, but luckily this never became a problem for me. I did sort of "freak out" at home and sprayed Lysol on every door handle and faucet. And I washed my hands repeatedly as if I were going into surgery.

Matt graduated with his master's in education just before Christmas, and his mom and brother came to spend some time with us. But Christmas was hard. I didn't want any gifts because I wasn't sure how long I would be around. I was also nervous about getting presents for the baby. I didn't want to jinx anything. Mostly, I was just thankful to have family around me, and I prayed that the baby and I would be healthy.

Just after Christmas, my hair started thinning. For me, hair loss was the hardest aspect of the entire ordeal. Don't get me wrong. Losing a breast is no picnic, but you can hide that. Your hair is a visible sign, and I had always had so much hair that my stylist had to thin it regularly. By New Year's, hair was coming out in clumps. I vowed that I would never complain about a bad hair day again!

My husband was an angel. I was eight months pregnant, bald, and had only one breast, but he made me feel beautiful with his constant reassurance.

Because it became too hard to handle questions about going through treatment while pregnant, I finally bought a wig. By then, I didn't have much hair left. I guess I thought I'd be one of the people who didn't lose hair, but with the drugs I was taking, it was a normal side effect. In retrospect, it would have been easier to shave my head instead of letting my hair fall out all over the shower—and the rest of the house, too. I toyed with the idea of becoming a blonde or a redhead, but in the end I bought a wig that was close to my normal hairstyle and color. I wore the wig in public, but mostly I wore scarves or went bald around the house.

The first day I wore the wig to work, I received several compliments on my cute haircut. It made me feel more confident. It also kept my head warm in the freezing winter temperatures.

With chemo appointments, blood checks, and visits to the obstetrician, I was in a doctor's office several times a week. I started seeing my obstetrician every two weeks after I was diagnosed, and then weekly, starting six weeks before my due date. She knew I was nervous about the effects of the chemo on the baby, so we scheduled several sonograms. I even saw a neonatologist for a Level II sonogram, which allowed a more in-depth look at the baby and a chance to screen for problems. My amniotic fluid was on the lower end of normal, but everything else looked great.

I never experienced nausea from my treatments. On some days I was more tired than usual and experienced some heartburn, but I never knew whether that came from chemotherapy, pregnancy, or a combination. The anti-nausea drugs available are amazing, and they are even prescribed for severe morning sickness during pregnancy. It made me feel better to know that what I was taking had been used by other pregnant women.

My college sorority sisters held a baby shower for me just before my last treatment. As I looked around the room at my friends, I thought, "Who would have imagined five years ago in college that we'd be sitting in a room filled with moms and children and that I would be in treatment for breast cancer?" All before our thirtieth birthdays.

My last chemotherapy treatment occurred on Wednesday, February 16, 2000. My oncologist called it "Graduation Day." Although he wanted me to have my blood counts checked during the next two weeks and then to see him once again for a check-up, this chapter in my life seemed to be almost over. I was ecstatic!

That evening, Matt, my mom, and I shared a casserole delivered by my P.E.O. sisters. We also celebrated our dog Haley's second birthday. My dad was out of town, but he and I chatted on the phone, also celebrating the end of my chemotherapy. I had five weeks until the baby was due and a list of projects for Matt to complete. I went to bed peacefully.

At 5:30 A.M. the next morning, my water broke. Matt and I were both frantic. How could I be in labor? I wasn't due for another five weeks. My obstetrician was on vacation. And I didn't have a bag packed. After rushing around pulling things together, we hurried to the hospital.

At the hospital, I asked whether we could stop my labor. "It's too early," I said.

"Honey, you're having a baby," replied the nurse.

Since this was my first child, we were told the baby probably wouldn't be delivered until the afternoon. Matt phoned my mom. I heard her squealing on the other end. We told her not to hurry, but she immediately called my dad so that he could travel home from a business trip a few hours away.

I was still tired from my treatment the day before, and as labor pains became more intense, I begged for an epidural. I have a low tolerance for pain anyway, and I wasn't prepared mentally for delivering so soon. Mom arrived at the hospital as I was sending Matt out for the second time to ask about an epidural. Finally, the anesthesiologist arrived and administered the shot. What a relief. Now the nurses had to tell me when I was having contractions.

I was wearing my wig at the beginning of hard labor, but it kept popping off, so finally I flung it across the room. The doctor on call joked that we had matching bald heads. Less than five hours after my water broke, I gave birth to a beautiful baby boy weighing 5 pounds, 1 ounce. And he had a full head of hair!

Matt and I both wept. I might be completely bald from the side effects of chemotherapy, but our son's full head of hair showed that the chemo had not affected him. It was like a sign from God.

Our little boy was beautiful and innocent, and I knew God had given him to me to help me through a very tough time. As hard as it was to endure treatment for cancer while pregnant, I often think the pregnancy helped me discover my tumor. And I know it kept me focused on staying healthy for both of us and for the future of our family together.

We debated all day over what to name the baby, finally choosing Parker Matthew. Parker was my mom's maiden name and Matthew was my husband's name, but it also means "Gift of God." All children are miracles, but Parker seemed to be a special gift.

Because Parker arrived five weeks early, we hadn't finished his nursery. We also didn't have a car seat in which to bring him home, so my dad and Matt went to pick one up. But the one they got wasn't the pattern I had wanted. Hormones took over, and I started crying. My oncologist stopped by and thought something awful had happened. When I explained, he looked dumbfounded—after all we'd had been through, I was worried about a car seat pattern? Still, my parents headed back to Babies-R-Us to get the right car seat.

As we left the hospital, our baby safe in his new car seat, I felt overwhelmed by life's goodness. Yes, I was bald, missing a breast, and hurting from just delivering a baby, but I was with my boys, ready to start a brand new chapter in our lives. My world was perfect.

Kim

My first day of chemotherapy was Valentine's Day. Happy Valentine's Day to me! Since my tumor was large (4 centimeters by 3 centimeters—a little smaller than a golf ball), and since the cells were dividing quickly and growing fast, my team of doctors decided on neo-adjuvant chemotherapy before surgery. The surgeon had already biopsied my lump, and I didn't have clean margins. If the mastectomy and reconstruction were done first, the oncologist would have to wait five to six weeks for me to recover before starting chemotherapy, and that was too long.

I was scheduled for four treatments of Adriamycin ("the red devil") and Cytoxan—one treatment every three weeks.

To ease my nerves before receiving my first round of chemotherapy, I started keeping a journal. I planned to e-mail it to family and friends so that they could share my experience. Four hours before my first chemotherapy infusion, I sat at my computer pounding out all my thoughts, fears, and feelings. As I wrote, I also decided to write a "Thought for the Week" and "Lessons I Am Learning from Breast Cancer."

My first thought came from Harry S. Truman: "A pessimist is one who makes difficulties of his opportunities, and an optimist is one who makes opportunities of his difficulties." Yes, I decided, that's how I'll handle this experience.

For my first lesson, I wrote this:

I am a person who is *living* with cancer, not dying from it. I refuse to let this experience take over my life. I am a mother, a wife, a daughter, a sister, a friend, a community activist, a political guru. I may have breast cancer, but breast cancer doesn't have me! I may not be able to be in control of the cancer, but I am in control of how I live my life, and I choose to make the most of each and every day God has given me. I'll take time to experience the good things that life offers.

I let Scott read the e-mail before I sent it. As he read, tears streamed down his face. Together, we hit the "send" button, and then we were off to chemotherapy.

As Scott and I waited for the oncology nurse to give us a crash course in Chemotherapy 101, Scott half-jokingly pointed to the view outside our window. "Not exactly uplifting," he whispered—we were across the street from a graveyard. We entered the infusion room with its circle of recliners and, like Patti, Jana, and Jen, I felt as if I'd entered a geriatric ward. I was by far the youngest person there.

Once you have lymph nodes removed, you are advised not to have blood draws or blood pressure taken on that arm because it is thought to increase the risk for lymphedema on that side. With one "good arm," it can be difficult to find a good vein. Apparently, from the get-go, my vein was hard to find. It took twenty minutes of hunting before the nurse could insert the IV.

First, I was given an anti-nausea drug. Then Adriamycin (Patti called it cherry Kool-Aid; it reminded me of red roses).

Next, Cytoxan. All in all, the treatment took about three hours, and Scott sat right beside me the entire time.

After my first treatment, Scott and I went to pick up Brandon from daycare. He came running to the car to give me a big hug. That made everything seem okay. I was tired initially and a little nauseated, but the anti-nausea drug worked; and though I slept most of the time for a week, and also felt nauseated, I did not throw up.

What was affected was my sense of smell, which increased threefold. I never knew there were so many bad colognes and perfumes. I went back to work after a week, and in the elevator, I had to hold my nose when we rode past the cafeteria. The special of the day was sauerkraut.

You learn who your true friends are when you're diagnosed with cancer. People I had not seen in years were now checking in weekly. My friend Crystal came over and cleaned the house. (You know you have a good friend when she comes and cleans your toilets.) Others brought meals. A fellow cancer survivor suggested that I have a friend or family member coordinate my meal and other needs, one of the best pieces of advice I received; my friend Kristin volunteered to do this for me.

As a firefighter, Scott worked twenty-four-hour shifts every third day. He was also the cook in our family. But on the days he worked, it was all I could do to make time for Brandon. For five months, Kristin coordinated the meals that were dropped off at our house every Monday, Wednesday, and Friday. It was an amazing and much-appreciated gesture of support.

My friends also decided that before I lost my hair they would throw me a hat party. Even though a mini-blizzard hit the area the day of the party, twenty friends bravely showed up, "hats in hand." Brandon, in giggly two-year-old fashion, tried on every hat while I took photos. He'll love them when he grows up.

After the hat party, eight of us had a slumber party at my friend Kristin's. It was like old times in the sorority house, and perfectly timed because my hair started falling out that very evening. I could actually pull it out in clumps, and with my friends there, it was kind of fun. I gave each one some of my hair as a souvenir.

On the Web site Scott had set up, I continued to post my journals, news updates, and pictures. My friends could also post notes in my guest book, and I enjoyed reading these. I especially appreciated the prayers, which became a strong part of my healing process. A sorority sister who had survived cancer several years before gave me a "Something for Jesus to Do" box. Whenever I had a problem I felt I couldn't handle, I put it in the box and let God do his work. The verse that came with the box read:

Good morning. I am the Lord your God. Today, I will be handling all of your problems. Please remember that I do not need your help. If the devil happens to deliver a situation to you that you cannot handle, DO NOT attempt to resolve it. Kindly put it in the "Something for Jesus to Do" box. It will be addressed in my time, not yours. Once the matter is placed in the box, do not hold onto it or attempt to remove it. Holding on or removal will delay the resolution of your problem. If it is a situation that you are capable of handling, please consult me in prayer to be sure that it is the proper resolution. Because I do not sleep nor do I slumber, there is no need for you to lose any sleep. Rest my child. If you need to contact me, I am only a prayer away. Love Eternally, The Lord Your God.

AUTHOR UNKNOWN

I was astounded at the wide readership of my journals. Every day, I received e-mails from people I didn't even know. My sorority posted my journals on their Web site, and sorority sisters from across the country sent me notes and cards. I'd valued my sorority experience while in college—now I was experiencing its lifelong benefits.

At one chemo treatment, I sat down beside another young woman. When we started talking, I learned that my e-mail journal had been forwarded to her. She was thirty-three, the mother of two children, and had just been diagnosed with cancer. This was her first chemo treatment. I knew how nervous and scared she felt (I'd been there!), so I tried to calm her fears as much as I could.

Another e-mail came from a friend who was at her hair salon talking about my experience when the salon's owner came over and showed her a stack of my journal entries. She had printed them out for a friend.

Also, I kept track of the number of women who started doing monthly breast self-examinations because of my story! By the end of a year, the number was nearing five hundred. I felt I was making a difference, and that kept me going.

Not by choice but by necessity, I kept working during treatment. I was a contract employee and had no disability insurance. I never realized its importance because—like most people at age thirty—I thought I was invincible. Fortunately, my treatment costs were covered because I was on Scott's health insurance plan. However, I could not afford to take off work for six months while undergoing treatment.

Luckily, my managers were very understanding and let me work from home part of the time. One boss was a breast cancer survivor herself, and the other's mother had recently been diagnosed. I truly believe that God had a hand in having me work there when I was diagnosed; the compassion and understanding from my managers made my life much easier.

Working during treatment was also a sort of therapy because it allowed me to focus on things other than my illness. There were days, however, when the chemo clouded my thinking. This phenomenon is called "chemo brain," and I was experiencing it firsthand.

There are many great support groups for breast cancer survivors, but at the one meeting I attended, I realized I was at a different place in my life than the other women. Many were retired, and most talked about their grandchildren, but I was thinking about my future, my career, my young son, and whether I would be able to have more children.

I found my own support group through Patti and the other Nordie Girls. Also, I came across the Young Survival Coalition (YSC) (www.youngsurvival.org), the only international organization focused on young women with breast cancer. On their Web site, I read about other young breast cancer survivors and found helpful tips on chemotherapy, side effects, and other issues. It helped to know I was not alone in my fight. Finding this organization was exactly what I needed.

During much of my treatment, the most difficult thing was not chemo's side effects, but being the mother of a two-year-old. Brandon had reached the terrible twos while I was undergoing chemotherapy—screaming fits and all.

And there was one "week from hell" that started with hair loss. When I got out of the shower one morning, the top of my head was almost bald. A few stringy pieces of hair hung from the sides. It looked horrible! Two hours later, I had to introduce a national speaker to two hundred women at a Madam President forum, so, with no time to get my head shaved, I resolutely put on one of my new black hats.

As I introduced the president of the Ms. Foundation for Women, I told the audience I had been diagnosed with breast cancer two months ago and realized now, more than ever, how important it was to become an advocate for women's issues. Talking about my experience empowered me.

That night, Scott, Brandon, and I went to get my head shaved. I was worried about Brandon's reaction. Would he know I was still his mommy? When Brandon felt my head with his hand, he smiled. I didn't have my head shaved smooth, but kept a little peach fuzz, which Brandon liked to pet as if I were a dog. I thought I would be much more upset about losing my hair, but I dealt with it pretty well. I also enjoyed not having to shave my legs or underarms. And the good news: Although my eyelashes and eyebrows thinned, they did not fall out completely.

The very next night, Scott and I had to have our Dalmatian, Bailey, put to sleep. Bailey had been a part of our family since he was a puppy; he even slept with Scott and me on the bed. Scott and I cried like babies. I had to keep telling myself that maybe God was trying to alleviate extra stresses in my life.

But that was not all. The day after we had Bailey put to sleep, Scott went to the emergency room, complaining of severe stomach pain. He had diverticulitis, a disease that occurs when small pouches in the colon become infected or inflamed. It occurs primarily in people older than fifty. "What's up with Scott and me, both getting diseases that occur usually in older people?" I wondered. The ER doc gave Scott antibiotics and told him to eat more fiber. In a few days, he was much better.

My "week from hell" led into my second round of chemo. I knew I'd feel tired, but expected no other side effects. Wrong! I started vomiting the day after the second treatment. My anti-nausea medicine was not working. New, stronger medicine also didn't work. For the next five days, I felt like crap, and for the first time since my ordeal started, I grew angry. I had to remind myself that things could be worse—I could have caught my cancer at a much later stage, or I could have contracted a different type, one for which the prognosis was not as good. Still, it was hard. One day, I was so tired that I had to crawl up the stairs.

When I felt better, I decided to do a little retail therapy. One day, while at the mall, my head got hot, so I decided to pull off my hat and went bald. I was amazed at the reactions. People equate baldness with sickness, so they feel uncomfortable. Actually, I felt free walking around hatless. I didn't mind being bald.

Besides my hats, I bought a wig—for $500—but I wore it only twice because it made my scalp itch; and not only that, Scott freaked out when he saw it. He preferred to see me bald, and I was comfortable with my new bald look.

My own lesson from all this? *It's just hair—it will grow back.* I am who I am, bald or not. After a while, I became so comfortable with my baldness that I took off my hat at meetings or when I ate. I even flaunted my cute little bald head when I gave presentations. In a way, baldness was my badge of courage. Not to mention that when I showed up, people noticed, which made my breast cancer awareness mission much easier. The sick part of me even used baldness a few times to get what I wanted when raising money for my favorite charities. People have a much harder time saying no when you're standing there with your bald head.

On my third round of chemo, I was late to my appointment. A friend had to talk me into going. I was tired of throwing up for a week, and now that I was feeling better, I didn't want to go through all that again. Not to mention that the steroids they gave me to take several days before my chemo treatment had me bouncing off the walls, and I felt great.

When I finished my fourth and final round of Adriamycin/ Cytoxan, I was so excited, and hopeful, too, that this would be my last treatment. That same day, I was chosen by a local magazine as of one of forty "Young Up-and-Coming Leaders." At the magazine photo shoot, I asked the photographer to take two shots: one with my hat and one without. They picked the hat shot for the magazine, but I'll cherish forever the photos of my bald head.

Being an activist while undergoing chemotherapy treatments was important to me. On the speaking circuit, I shared my story and urged early detection. For the Komen Race for the Cure, I sponsored a team with another friend and survivor. I'd participated in the race in the past, but seeing all those pink survivor shirts now had new meaning. I was one!

Here's another lesson I learned: While undergoing chemotherapy, it is important to take advantage of the time when you feel good to get as much stuff done as possible. But learn to say no. I'd been working on that before I had cancer; now I was forced to master the behavior. It was difficult. I've always been an organized, by-the-book type of person, good at taking care of life's details. Now I was learning not to sweat the small stuff. Time is a precious gift. I realized that I must use it as such and focus my energy on what's really important: my family, my friends, and work that I am passionate about. As I explained in a journal entry: "For now, my house may be dirty, I may not have my thank-you notes finished, I may misspell a few words [I had sent out a journal entry with a misspelled word and was appalled], and I may not return phone calls within a twenty-four-hour period, but that's okay because I am living life!"

I had my breast surgery after my first four rounds of chemotherapy, and shortly thereafter I had a Port-a-Cath surgically placed. This device enabled me to receive chemo treatments and have blood drawn without having to have a needle poked into my arm or hand each time.

A few months later, I'd recovered enough from the mastectomy with TRAM flap reconstruction to start another four rounds of chemotherapy (Taxotere). Although I had no lymph node involvement, based on my age and the size and aggressive nature of my tumor, the doctors wanted to play it safe. I wasn't happy to do chemo again, but I reacted much better to the Taxotere—I did have a brief allergic reaction, fatigue and diarrhea—but it was much more bearable.

My hair was a different story. Because I'd gone two months without chemo (due to surgery), it had started to grow back and was coming in darker. (Since I'd been highlighting it for so many years, who knows what my natural color really was?) After the second round of Taxotere, my new hair started to thin. I would rather have been bald. The in-between stage was not a pretty picture. Strangers probably thought I went to a really bad hairdresser.

At my eighth and final chemo treatment, the nurses presented me with a "Graduation Certificate." My Nordie's friends had balloons and candy waiting for me as well. But I was scared. For ten months, I'd had constant care, and I had fought with everything I had. Once they unhooked that last IV bag and sent me on my way, I felt as if they were waving a magic wand and saying, "Now you're cured." But there are no guarantees or "cure" for breast cancer. At least when I was being treated, I was killing the cancer. But now what?

As I left the doctor's office, I went to my car and cried and cried. What would the future hold for me?

CHAPTER SIX

A New
Sense of Normal

— Nordie's Café —
November 2002

hile Kim and Jen were settling into the corner booth, Jana waited for her special-order panini and told Patti what happened during her infusion the previous week. While still hooked up to the IV, she had seen a nurse give a patient a Certificate of Completion because it was her last day of chemotherapy. "This must be a new practice at the clinic—I never got a certificate!" she exclaimed. Patti and Jen nodded. This was indeed something new. Kim received a certificate at the end of her treatment, a couple of years after Patti, Jana, and Jen completed their treatments.

"I remember my oncologist calling it 'Graduation Day' and I was thrilled to reach that point, but I was also scared to be on my own," Jen noted. "I was so used to seeing at least one of my doctors every week during pregnancy that it was hard to let go of that connection."

"I was scared, too," admitted Kim.

Patti agreed. "It was like 'Okay, now you have completed your treatments. Say good-bye to your nurses and hope you never see them again.' What I really wanted was a card that declared, 'Congratulations, You're Cured!' Instead, the end of chemo was anticlimactic."

The others agreed.

Jana continued, "Milestones in life usually warrant some sort of celebration. Even a first-time driver gets an actual license. So in that sense, I think it's nice that the nurses are now giving out chemo completion certificates. But even more useful would be instructions on how to get your life back to normal!"

"But will our lives ever be 'normal' again?" asked Jen. "I have a new sense of normal. I changed after facing my own mortality and battling through cancer. I also became a first-time mom. It's a little hard to know which brought about the most change for me—fighting cancer or giving birth."

Kim concurred: "Becoming a mom was definitely life-changing, but so was battling and beating cancer, and it taught me lessons that I wouldn't change for anything in the world."

So at this luncheon we decided to share our perception of our own "new sense of normal."

Patti

I remember my last chemotherapy appointment much better than the treatment itself. I went to the oncologist's office three weeks after my last experience with Adriamycin and Cytoxan. I got my blood tests, set up a three-month follow-up appointment, and had an uneventful talk with my doctor about my decision not to go with Tamoxifen. And then just like that . . . she sent me off, proclaiming me "done."

"Being done" was the goal I had been single-mindedly pursuing, but I found the finish line confusing. When you finish a race, you get Gatorade; when you finish finals in college, you go to the bars. When you accomplish a large life goal, you buy yourself a piece of Swarovski crystal (at least if you're me). But what exactly do you do when you're sent home supposedly "cancer free"? My oncologist seemed like Tinkerbell. She "dinged" me with her magic wand, proclaimed me "healthy," and said, "Go back to life as you know it."

Only I couldn't. I wasn't the same person I'd been eight months earlier. While it was happening, I plowed through treatment, planning to pick up right where I had left off. I didn't consciously let cancer change me; but it did. I was different.

What didn't change in my new "normal"?

I continued to celebrate the presence of family and friends in my life. I celebrated weddings, anniversaries, and births; I traveled and I went to housewarmings. I continued to be a godmother to many pets, lavishing treats and hugs whenever I visited them at friends' homes. It would take months for my friends to un-teach their pets what I had so graciously taught them: "It's okay to sit on the new couch"; "Feel free to eat the whole bag of treats and then whine for more"; and "Yes, you do deserve more attention."

My dating life stayed dynamic. I remained proficient at turning down guys who drove Mustangs, which, in itself, is a valuable life skill. I was also granted the gift of dating my third Chris. My parents now referred to them by number—like orders from McDonald's. At any rate, a girl's gotta be thankful that there are still good men out there. I wasn't moving toward marriage, but I knew that my wedding gift to all my friends would be one very large, fun party.

At work, I continued to be promoted, to receive performance review ratings in the top 5 percent, and to build mentoring relationships. I knew the track to partner by heart, and I considered either working as a traveling consultant or making a move to my firm's Chicago office to make it happen faster. I knew where I was headed and I didn't intend to be slow in getting there.

With my energy back, I became involved in my company's participation in the local Corporate Challenge—an Olympic-style competition in which several corporations compete against each other in athletic events. I competed in track and field, basketball, and volleyball. Less than two years after finishing chemo, I completed my first triathlon (taking first in my division: a field of one). I also completed various runs, including the Komen Race for the Cure.

I cochaired my firm's March of Dimes Walk America team. Overall, I felt good about my professional life.

When I look back over my e-mails, I see that I can liken my new "normal" to a drink. It's this:

- *One part friends and family:* I just took a trip to St. Louis to help Melanie, my sorority sister, celebrate her engagement. I got a speeding ticket along the way, but what else is new?
- *One part work and travel:* I worked overtime for a couple of weeks and had no trouble doing that. Also made it to a baseball game and took a free trip to Los Angeles. I took a trip to Myrtle Beach for the Fourth of July weekend.
- *Half a part boyfriends:* He (my first Chris) got a new job in Dallas. He now finds good humor in singing "All my Ex's Live in Texas" to me on the phone. Where do I find these guys? (Chris #2 had moved to Dallas a year earlier; Chris #3 is stuck in Los Angeles.)

These parts of my life didn't change—but I was changed.

Postchemo life added a few more ingredients to my "life drink":

- *One part deeper understanding that some things in life are beyond my control*
- *A pinch of coping skills for dealing with the uncontrollable*
- *A taste in the back of my throat reminding me that the cancer could return*

Part of my new sense of normal can be explained by how challenging it was for me to deal with the fact that during my chemotherapy I was physically unable to do some things that I used to do with ease.

During chemotherapy, I volunteered to be part of my company's Corporate Challenge team by being a line judge for the volleyball competition. It seemed like a noble idea on my part. Since I couldn't play, I could at least be part of the team by providing support. I showed up and did a great job of line judging for my teams, but I had a sick feeling in my stomach the whole time.

During high school, I was a member of several teams: swimming, basketball, volleyball, and softball. And rarely did I ride the bench. I'd always figured that the stats people didn't want to play, or lacked the skill to play. I was always a player. When I served as line judge, I got a taste of what it felt like to "ride the bench." I didn't like it.

I didn't like it because riding the bench was beyond my control, and I've always had trouble handling things outside my control. I always believed that I could "work a little harder" to play more or "practice a little more" to play better. I could make things go my way. If cancer has taught me nothing else, it's that sometimes things were just beyond my control.

At the Corporate Challenge, I realized I couldn't be a spectator for a sport in which I'd once been a good team player. I'm too competitive. I love sports competition, but *only* as a participant. I looked for someone to fill my spot as a line judge, and, thankfully, a guy was hanging out watching a friend play. He graciously stepped in for me.

Then I needed a self-esteem booster. *Fast.* Something I could do physically to help me overcome feeling like a limp noodle.

I drove to the nearest swimming pool and threw down a quick 1,300-meter swim. That helped because I realized that, with or without fins, and with or without cancer, I could probably still wax just about anyone at the pool.

My new sense of normal, then, included a strategy for dealing with things beyond my control. First, admit when I'm not in control. Second, remedy the situation (in the example of being a line judge, it meant leaving). Third, do something to counter faltering self-esteem. This strategy empowered me and helped me be thankful for the things I could do and did have, instead of regretting what I couldn't do and didn't have.

When the chemo was finished, challenging my body physically was at the top of my list. I maintained a healthy lifestyle and added new energy to work and relationships. But my experience with cancer forced me to accept some limitations. Fear that I wasn't ready to acknowledge stirred within me. In my return to normal, I had to cope with these realities and understand that they would be as much a part of my life as Donna's dogs and cherry limeade.

My new normal included a scary six-month check-up and the celebration of my first cancer-free year. It also included regular check-ups and blood work, which interrupted work days with a nagging question: "Could this happen to me again?"

Jana

After four months of fighting cancer, my new-found freedom seemed uncomfortable at first. All my attention had been focused on getting through the challenges of surgery and chemotherapy. Now, what used to be normal felt foreign. I had to redefine my new sense of self.

I also had to adapt to a new routine. While treating and fighting my cancer, I had a plan, and I followed it by going into the clinic every week. Now, my safety net and routine were gone and I had to find other activities to fill my time. Of course, I had a wedding to pull off and a new life to begin with Chris. And I planned to return to work after my wedding. Beyond that, I took life one day at a time. For a while, my "normal" meant that nothing was the same as before and that I was uncertain of the future.

I noticed a change in mindset. Having a serious illness at a young age compresses what would ordinarily come from years of life experience into a much shorter time. I had stared death in the face. Now I knew that death could come knocking on my door at any time. I realized that I have little control over the length of my life.

I'm not afraid of death because I believe I am going to a better place, one called "heaven." In heaven, I believe there will be no suffering, pain, or illness. Wondering what my final days on earth will be like became part of my new "normal." These were thoughts I didn't have before cancer.

Now it's normal for me to worry about the loneliness Chris will feel the first night he spends in bed alone without me. I have had to come to terms with what would make him happy when I'm gone. We believe we are each other's soulmates, and I can't stand the thought of being "replaced." But I also know that Chris is meant to be a husband; therefore, if being a husband to someone else after I'm gone will make him happy, then he should get remarried.

As newlyweds, Chris and I made sure that our wills and other legal affairs were settled, but when we went to sign the papers, the day didn't feel normal at all. It was difficult to make sure, at the age of twenty-seven, that I had a durable power of attorney. It was strange to decide at such an early age who would inherit my "estate."

My way of interacting with others and my perception of how others viewed me also changed. My new sense of normal included a distrust of my body. After all, it had seemingly failed me by getting cancer and then rejecting chemotherapy.

I panicked every time I got a headache, a bellyache, or a new red spot on my hand that looked like vasculitis. Chris suggested I "talk to someone." So now my sense of normal included paying a professional to listen to me as I rattled off my fears and to help me realize that my body is strong and becoming stronger and is not failing me. I still go in for what I call "booster" therapy sessions at least four times a year. That's my normal now.

It also became normal to toss the Victoria's Secret catalogues in the trash rather than circling things for Chris to order for me. My new normal is putting a breast prosthesis (a.k.a. my "fake boob") in my bra every day and taking it out each night. Washing it to keep it clean. And making sure it air dries in a safe place. Once, one—or both—cats took a big bite out of my fake boob when I left it on the counter overnight.

My mental checklist before I leave the house now goes like this: "Iron off? Check. Cats accounted for? Check. Teeth brushed? Check. Fake boob in my bra? Check. Doors locked? Check."

For several months, while my hair grew out, donning a wig for work became another part of my daily routine. On windy winter days, I worried that my wig would fly off my head in the parking lot. But at work, I chose to deal with wig issues rather than with bald issues. At home, I immediately traded my wig for my comfy chicken cap.

For a full year after chemotherapy, I did not feel like "myself." I quit reading several fashion magazines I used to enjoy. Women with two breasts adorn their pages. The fact that I'd had cancer and lost a breast was part of my new normalcy, and seeing the breasts highlighted on every page reminded me of how abnormal I felt. Only recently have I begun to enjoy these magazines again.

It became normal to go to bed earlier, the polar opposite from my life before cancer, when I burned the candle at both ends. Also, I suffered from chemo brain. My head was cloudy from the poisons that were put in my body. The symptoms included memory loss and feelings of stress. To this day, I still have occasional chemo brain moments, and I have accepted this will always be "normal" for me.

My new normal also includes frequent medical follow-ups. Every three months, I visit my doctors for tests. Every six months, I go for a CT scan and a bone scan. Before each test, I get cranky. I am scared of hearing "We have found cancer in your [fill in the blank]." Going to the doctor has forever changed for me.

And then there is the problem of describing the status of my cancer. Should I say I "have" cancer or I "had" cancer? I believe you're not supposed to say you have "had" cancer until you reach the magical five years after diagnosis without incident. Then you can say you are in remission. Some people use the term "remission" the second they have had their mastectomies. Others use it at the end of chemotherapy. And still others, like me, think waiting a full five years before proclaiming themselves officially in remission is most accurate.

So, for me, my normal is that I have a disease and I will have it for the rest of my life; in that sense it's much like a chronic illness such as diabetes. It requires constant attention, follow-up, and flexibility. That's just the way it will have to be for me—my new normal.

I have learned that "normal" is whatever I want it to be. It is reprioritizing things in my life. I take my spiritual life more seriously now, and, like Patti, I learned the importance of tithing and striving for agape love. And though I love my work, I now take as many vacations as possible. My life is family and friends, work and fun. It is not being afraid to die and not being afraid to live. Like the little guy on my cap, I repeat the mantra "Life is good"—even on days when life may seem bad, because, after all, I'm alive!

Jen

The end of treatment was both exciting and terrifying, much like riding a roller coaster. I was thrilled to be finished with chemotherapy and to think about my hair growing back, but I had lost trust in my body's ability to fight anything that might be lurking. I had also received so much attention from my doctors, family, and friends that when it ended abruptly, I felt a bit alone. Suddenly, I was supposed to move past this episode and go back to life the way it used to be. That was impossible, so I had to find my own new sense of normal.

Three weeks after my last chemotherapy treatment, I marched back to the oncologist's office for my post-treatment check-up, only this time, I brought Parker—who was a tiny newborn! As I waited for my appointment, I realized I was nervous about no longer coming in every week for blood checks or treatments. I thought about my pathology report, which indicated that my tumor was estrogen-negative and only slightly progesterone-positive. This meant I was not a good candidate for hormone therapy, such as Tamoxifen, unlike Patti and Jana. Because their tumors were positive for estrogen and progesterone (ER/PR +), hormone therapy may have helped reduce the risk of a recurrence for them.

However, I was strongly HER2 positive. Approximately 25 percent of women with breast cancer are HER2 positive, meaning they have an excess of a protein known as HER2, and this makes the cancer spread quickly. When my oncologist first reviewed my pathology report with me, he remarked that he hoped he never had to treat me again, but that there was a promising new drug on the market for women who are HER2 positive. This drug is called Herceptin, and although I knew that being positive was an unfavorable prognostic factor, it was good news to know that there is a drug that can help me, should my cancer ever spread. I asked whether there was a clinical trial so that I could take Herceptin then—to prevent my cancer from spreading. But at the time, it was only approved for the treatment of metastatic breast cancer. There were trials for early stage breast cancer patients going on at the time, but I would have qualified for them only if I had had lymph node involvement. It haunted me that I could not give my body the extra treatment, but it also comforted me to know that there was a treatment available should my cancer return.

My first two years out of treatment found me seeing my oncologist every three months, my surgeon every six months. Anticipating each appointment or medical test left me feeling anxious about what they might find. My oncologist consoled me by saying that if I was not showing symptoms, he wasn't likely to find anything else, either. And I have found that the further out I am from my diagnosis and treatments, the less I worry. In fact, this year, I almost forgot to schedule my annual check-up with the oncologist until my mom mentioned it! Although it felt liberating not to be so anxious, it was also a little scary for me to realize that I seemed to be taking things for granted.

Since I was a new mom as well as a cancer survivor, my new normal included caring for a baby. After three months of maternity leave, I returned to work, and that was hard, but I didn't have the option of staying home. I couldn't give up my health and life insurance benefits, and we needed my salary.

Matt was off all summer, so Parker did not start full-time daycare until he was six months old. Knowing that my son was at home with Matt made my first days back at work more tolerable for me. Sometimes, especially during team meetings, I would think about how caught up in the rituals of work people become. They forget to take a step back and recognize what's really important.

I enjoyed my career, but after becoming a mom, I learned to work smarter. I feel most fulfilled being with my family and staying active in breast cancer causes.

As part of my new normal, I also decided to take better care of my body. I've always been on the thin side, so I never needed to work out to manage my weight. But now I joined the gym at work: I attended yoga classes, lifted weights, and did cardio. The yoga classes were physically and mentally refreshing.

I also paid more attention to the food I ate, eating broccoli and Brussels sprouts as often as I could for their proclaimed cancer-fighting properties. I even tried to start eating chicken, which I had long detested. I still eat the occasional French fry, and sometimes I drink a glass of wine, but I think more about what goes into my body. By having chemotherapy at such a young age, I now face other potential long-term health issues such as osteoporosis and heart disease. I simply remind myself that I will be happy to live long enough to deal with these issues if they ever arise, but I do want to make sure that I do whatever I can now by keeping my body as healthy as possible.

As my body started returning to its prepregnancy weight and shape (but I'm kidding myself—I know my body will never be quite the same again!), the loss of my breast became more of a reality. I didn't wear low-cut clothes before, but now I had to be extra careful when I bent over so that Boobsie (the name I had given my prosthesis) would not escape from my bra. And swimsuit weather was coming! It is difficult enough to shop for swimsuits, but trying to find a cute mastectomy swimsuit designed for a fifty- or sixty-year-old was frustrating and humiliating for me. I still had decent-looking legs, and I didn't want a skirted swimsuit. Finally, I had a pocket sewn into a regular swimsuit. It looked pretty good, but summer lit the fire of my desire to have reconstructive surgery.

Six months after Parker was born, I looked more seriously at reconstructive surgery. A TRAM flap would give me a tummy tuck, but I hoped to have another child, so I was afraid that procedure would be a waste. An expander, followed by an implant, was unappealing because I had high hopes of breast-feeding next time. To make things worse, the surgeon said that if I kept my natural breast, it might need to be reduced and lifted to match the implant. (Nothing like having a droopy boob in your twenties.) I wasn't interested in being smaller in the chest area, either. In the end, I decided to put reconstruction on my to-do list as a five-year-mark gift to myself.

I could have lived without my breast. With clothes on, no one could tell. But I'd grown tired of dealing with the breast prosthesis, and I wanted to feel sexier for myself and for Matt. As much as I loved our intimate times, the scar on my chest made me feel unattractive. For him, it was never an issue, but I could not get over it. As much as I hate to admit it, I needed my breast to feel sexy again. The decision to undergo reconstruction is a personal one, and the procedure is not right for everyone.

In deciding which option to pursue, I did a lot of soul searching. A TRAM flap would be nice, especially for the bonus of a tummy tuck after pregnancy. But I was worried about breast cancer on the opposite side and I did not have enough fat to make two new breasts. Because I was so young at the time of my original diagnosis, my risk for developing breast cancer later in life is greater than that of women who have never had the disease.

Removing a completely healthy breast might seem extreme, but I knew it would greatly reduce the risk of more cancer. I thought about genetic testing to help make the final decision, but I knew I was already at high risk. My mom's sister, brother, and father had all been diagnosed with cancer. Something was going on in our family.

Like Jana, I chose to have a prophylactic mastectomy on the right breast and have bilateral reconstruction with saline implants. My first surgery took place in the summer because that is when Matt would be able to take care of the home front. The pre-op waiting area brought back a flood of memories from nearly five years before. This time, though, I was choosing to have surgery.

On the day of my first surgery, our pastor came and prayed with us. Then my plastic surgeon marked my chest, and off I went. Because my two surgeons worked at the same time, the procedure was completed in only two hours.

Nothing looked suspicious (i.e., cancerous), and after a night in the hospital, I went home. I was delighted to wake up with two small mounds on my chest from the 75 cubic centimeters of saline placed in my expanders. The best news of all was that nothing bad was found during my surgery.

Two weeks later, I had my first fill. I took a Valium an hour before the appointment to relax my muscles. The doctor used a device with a magnet in it to find my ports so that he could fill the expanders with saline solution (90 cubic centimeters). Matt held my hand and was amazed to watch the mounds grow right in front of his eyes. When I sat up, I felt pressure in my chest. I was sore, but also in awe of what was taking place in my body. It took me three days to recover from that first fill. I decided to have three more fills, each with 75 cubic centimeters instead of

90. I returned to work with two fills to go, and I wondered how my coworkers would respond to my "growing" process. Those who knew were very supportive, and I doubt that anyone else even noticed. All in all, it took four visits to get "the girls," as Jana called them, fully inflated.

After the fills were complete, I put on a normal bra for the first time in nearly five years! It was such an amazing feeling. I had cleavage again. My breasts were rock hard, but they looked great. Actually, I didn't need to wear a bra. My new breasts were perky! When I asked the nurse whether they would ever droop, she said, "No, you and Matt will be in a nursing home some day and you'll be the only one there with perky boobs!"

For the first time after my surgery, I felt comfortable putting on lingerie. Now that I could fill out both sides, I felt sexy again. My self-esteem was returning as well as my desire to be intimate.

During my next surgery, the expanders were replaced with implants. Implants would be softer and the plastic surgeon would adjust "the girls" to make them as close to the same size as possible. The surgery was scheduled to last an hour, so my mom grew pretty nervous when an hour and a half went by, but my surgeon had simply spent some extra time perfecting the girls. Recovering from this surgery was much easier than it had been when the expanders were put in.

I debated about whether to finish the "girls" with nipples and areolas. In the end, I decided I would go all out and have them look as close to the real thing as possible. The procedure would also help hide the scar line. Six weeks after the implants, I went for nipple creation. I was awake and talking to my surgeon the entire time as he cut and twisted my existing scar line to form a nipple on each breast. Nipples definitely made them feel more like breasts. They were very perky at first, but have since gone down.

The final step was the tattooing of the areolas. This was oddly fun and stressful at the same time. We were starting from scratch, and there were numerous nipple colors to choose from. From a pink shade, similar to the color of my nipples before I became pregnant, the spectrum moved to the brownish color they turned after pregnancy. I opted for a shade in the middle. This final step made the reconstruction process feel complete. I never imagined I would get a tattoo, and now I had two!

For my five-year mark, I made three goals for myself: I wanted to run (not walk) my first Race for the Cure and raise $5,000 for the local race to commemorate this milestone. I also wanted to have my reconstruction completed. True to my word, I raised more than $5,000 that year. I didn't run in the race, though, because I was in the middle of the reconstruction process. Still, I was proud to have accomplished two out of three goals.

As part of my new normal, I also became a breast cancer advocate and tried to help other women facing a breast cancer diagnosis. In October 2000, my employer sponsored a breast cancer awareness campaign. I helped implement the campaign, and I was chosen as the company's corporate "Speak Out Ambassador." It was very empowering for me to move from cancer patient to "survivor spokesperson." I was flown to New York, where I met the *Today Show* team and was interviewed on the *Early Show,* and I also appeared on several other New York and local television stations. I loved promoting a cause so near and dear to my heart.

I also began to speak at colleges and for alumni events through the Ribbons of Pink Foundation. When I was twenty,

someone gave a talk about her mom's experience with breast
cancer. I never imagined that in just seven years I, too, would
be speaking about cancer. Because I found my lump through
breast self-examination, I emphasize the importance of this
routine when I speak.

The support I received meant so much to me. I wanted to
"pay it forward," so I looked for ways to help women who
would "one day wear my bra" as I heard Lillie Shockney, ad-
ministrative director of the Johns Hopkins Avon Foundation
Breast Center describe it.

I started volunteering with the American Cancer Society's
Reach to Recovery program. It provides one-on-one peer coun-
seling for women diagnosed with breast cancer by matching
them to similarly diagnosed women. I also respond to phone
calls from my surgeon, friends, and coworkers looking for support. Sometimes I feel it does me more good than it does them,
but ultimately I hope it helps them to see that Parker and I both
survived this terrifying situation.

A month after treatment ended, I was invited to a breast
cancer survivor luncheon sponsored by the Komen Foundation. As I walked into the hotel lobby, I ran into Jana. We immediately recognized each other from high school. We had
heard about each other, but had never put two and two together because our last names had changed with marriage.

It was wonderful to meet another twenty-something survivor. But when she told me she'd had a recurrence, I went
numb. She was facing my greatest fear. Though she told me
that her tumor was smaller than mine and that it had no lymph
node involvement, I was terrified. I reminded myself that many
other women were doing great, years after diagnosis.

Jana told me about her chemo friend Patti. She and Patti were both undergoing treatments for recurrences, although Patti's case was more severe. Patti was going to be honored at the Ribbons of Pink event and, since I was volunteering, I would meet her. And when I did, I knew she was a firecracker. By this time, her cancer had spread to her lungs, liver, and bones, but she was living as though this were a mere inconvenience rather than a life-threatening event. I was in awe of her zest for life.

People ask how far out I am from my breast cancer. There are so many anniversaries. My initial diagnosis that forever changed my life. My surgery date: the day I lost my breast. The happiest anniversary was the end of chemotherapy because it marked the beginning of my life as a "survivor." It's easy to remember that date because it's exactly one day before Parker's birthday.

Another part of my new normal was learning to accept the label of breast cancer "survivor." I didn't like the implication that only women who outlive the disease are survivors. I think the courage that women show, even those who die from the disease, makes them survivors, too. But that's what I am: "A Survivor."

Kim

I had finished all my treatments. The doctors waved their magic wands and sent me on my merry way. Now I was supposed to forget all this stuff and get back to a normal life. To the outside world and to family and friends, I had beaten the disease, my hair was coming back, and I looked as normal as I did before. However, I was not the same person.

Cancer changed me, and, in my opinion, for the better. I learned more about myself and others through my diagnosis and treatments. I called on strengths I didn't know I had. I had to look deep within myself, and I found more empathy, openness, happiness, honesty, toughness, grit, and perspective. I learned that life is precious and fragile; in spite of the pain and tears, my cancer diagnosis became one of the most enriching experiences of my life. I realized that my family and friends are the most important treasures in life and that I should not take them for granted.

In the first months after completing chemotherapy, I enjoyed doing the simple things that I never thought I would say I enjoyed—such as going to the grocery store and running errands. It felt so good to be able to do these things without becoming totally exhausted.

A month after "Graduation Day," I watched an Oprah show that focused on breast cancer during Breast Cancer Awareness Month. I had not had the time or the energy to think fully about what I'd gone through. Oprah's show featured several young women who talked about their treatments, their hopes, and their fears. As I watched those women talk about chemotherapy treatments, being wheeled into surgery, going bald, and their desires to be around to raise their children, I realized that they were me. I started bawling. I cried my eyes out. It was as if I saw myself and what I had been through for the very first time.

A few weeks later, the harsh reality of living with breast cancer really hit me. My right hand (the side on which I'd had surgery) started to swell. I learned I had lymphedema, which is a potential risk for anyone who has had lymph nodes removed and/or radiation to an area where there is a prevalence of lymph nodes. The body's lymphatic system removes extra protein and water from body tissues and returns them to the blood system. A damaged lymphatic system may disrupt these pathways. Chronic symptoms require specialized treatment.

Lymphedema can occur a few months or a few years after surgery and, if left untreated, causes a lot of pain and damage. I now wear a compression sleeve and glove when I exercise, fly, or engage in strenuous activity. The arm must be kept spotlessly clean and I must avoid any type of heavy lifting or repetitive movement (so I guess vacuuming is out!). I still pick up Brandon, even though he weighs 45 pounds. I have to wear gloves while doing housework, gardening, or any work that could result in even a minor injury. I have to avoid cutting my cuticles, and I am supposed to use an electric razor when I shave under my right arm, although I refuse to do this.

Some days, I feel like wrapping my right hand and arm in germ-free bubble wrap and never using it again. However, even though I don't want to have sausage fingers for the rest of my life, I'll take sausage fingers over the alternative any day. What does make it difficult is that every time I look at my hand, it reminds me that I had breast cancer. Still, I have learned to accept my lymphedema and I don't let it stop me from living or from doing the things I love. I just try to make wise choices.

My new sense of normal taught me the reality of chemo brain. Sometimes I'll do or say something for which there is no explanation. And my memory is not as good as it used to be. I've asked other survivors how long I can use the chemo brain excuse, and they all say for the rest of my life. So until I can blame my forgetfulness on old age, I'll blame it on chemo brain.

My new sense of normal also taught me that beauty comes from within and that there is much more to me than my physical appearance. I learned to love my new body. I have my battle scars, but with each year, they are fading. I still have my flat tummy. If I decide to have more children, we'll see how that affects the TRAM flap reconstruction.

I am also happy to report that my hair has come back. My hair originally came back dark and curly. I'm a blonde at heart, so thank goodness for that bottle of color. And yes, even the hair on my arms and legs came back, so I now have to shave again—a mixed blessing!

Mostly, my new sense of normal means living every day to the fullest. I like to think I kicked breast cancer's butt and will live until I'm ninety. But, in reality, none of us knows. I could step outside tomorrow and be hit by a bus. For me, life is about now—today. Today is the only guarantee I have, so I am making it count.

Before cancer, I was always concerned about my life plan: my five-year plan, my ten-year plan, and my retirement plan. I had my entire life mapped out. Then I got breast cancer. It taught me that we're not in control. Instead of worrying about everything, we need to worry only about the things we do have control over. As for the rest, I give it up to God or put it in my "Something for Jesus to Do" box.

In my life, after breast cancer, I choose to view the glass as half full. Life is about choices. One of my favorite quotes comes from Father Alfred Souza. He said, "For a long time it had seemed to me that life was about to begin—real life. But there was always some obstacle in the way, something to be gotten through first, some unfinished business, time still to be served, and a debt to be paid. Then life would begin. At last it dawned on me that these obstacles were my life."

Everyone encounters bumps in the road of life. We can react one of two ways: We can feel sorry for ourselves, be angry, and spend all our energy asking why. Or we can take control of how we react, accept that obstacles are a part of life, and be happy anyway. Life is about choices. As part of my new normal, I choose to be happy.

CHAPTER SEVEN

Can It Happen to Me . . . Again???

—— *Nordie's Café* ——
December 2002

It was New Year's Eve, and we were all in a festive mood. Patti was beaming because her brother, David, was in town. She talked about going to her friend Donna's house for the evening. "We're just going to hang out, watch movies, and have a sleepover. It's going to be great!"

Jen and Matt had plans as well. "Parker is staying with his grammy and granddad tonight," Jen said. "For once, we actually have New Year's plans and are spending it with college friends."

After lunch, Kim was going to her parents' house in mid-Missouri with Brandon and Scott for some holiday fun. Jana looked forward to taking it easy and staying home for New Year's with Chris.

Even though we all had vastly different plans for the evening, we were happy to see each other and we looked forward to the New Year.

Today we spoke about the dreaded "R" word, "recurrence," the topic of the next chapter in our evolving book. Every cancer survivor fears being told his or her cancer has come back. As Kim neared her one-year cancer anniversary, she constantly thought about whether her cancer might return. Even though Jen was more than three years out, she was still nervous at the thought of a recurrence. And unfortunately for Patti and Jana, they both knew firsthand about cancer recurrence. The "R" word had crept into both their lives since their original diagnoses.

Kim and Jen admired Patti and Jana for their remarkable attitudes toward their recurrences. Although Patti and Jana both insisted that the treatments were an inconvenience that interfered with their lives, it was an inconvenience they simply lived with. After all, the additional treatments were saving their lives!

Once again, our monthly luncheon was a catharsis for all of us. Although our respective experiences were unique, many things about them overlapped. We shared our anxiety about upcoming tests, and we were thrilled when one of us had good results. And we were devastated when one of us had a setback or received bad news.

As always, the time passed too quickly. We hugged each other good-bye and looked forward to wonderful things in the new year, including, of course, our lunches at Nordie's.

Patti

You feel as though you had hiked the highest mountain, conquered the Roman Empire, and jumped through every hoop placed in your way when your cancer is pronounced "gone." But still, every time you enter a hospital or a doctor's office to get a "routine" set of tests, fear haunts the back of your mind. It's not so much the annual "feel-up" from the doctor that puts you ill at ease. (I always picture that scene in *Sixteen Candles* where they say, "Look, she's gotten her boobies," and that cracks me up.) It's more the excruciating week after a blood test, mammogram, or precautionary ultrasound while you wait for the results.

I had a scare about six months after my initial surgery. My surgeon felt something in my nonreconstructed breast and, "just to be cautious," wanted me to get an ultrasound. Was it a lumpy breast, scar tissue from my breast reduction, or—horror of horrors—the return of cancer? When she asked whether it bothered me to get a precautionary test, I responded with false confidence: "Shoot, what's the worst you could tell me? That I have breast cancer?" We both giggled at the small chance that this could be the outcome. Happily, the ultrasound results came back negative.

I was living under a false pretense: I thought that since I'd taken all the precautionary measures the first time, it could not happen to me a second time. But it did. After an active summer, approximately a year and a half after my surgery, when I had completed my first triathlon, had worked more than 1.5 persons' worth of overtime, and had hauled six laptops from site to site so that I could offer computer training, my back began to hurt. I thought I had injured it hauling laptops, but the physical therapy I was doing for pain didn't seem to help. In fact, the pain was getting worse. I couldn't jog on my trip to Chicago. I couldn't sleep on the uncomfortable hotel beds without massive efforts to un-kink my back the next morning.

It was after I went in for my routine blood tests that I got "the call." As usual, I was multitasking on my way to pick up test results, and I was running late. On the way, I got two phone calls from the doctor's office asking whether I planned to make it to my appointment. The second time, I was two blocks away, and I almost snapped at the receptionist.

Didn't she know I was driving forty-five minutes out of my way from work to get blood tests that would give the same results as always? Then suddenly the realization hit me: They wouldn't be so concerned unless there was something I needed to hear in person. I had tried to call in for my test results twenty minutes after the first phone call, but they wouldn't give me the results over the phone.

I drove the last two blocks in silence and prayer. Suddenly, I wanted someone with me. I didn't want to hear this news, whatever it was, alone. It was the middle of the morning. I hadn't told anyone about the blood test. After all, it was routine. Just the month before, at my oncologist's office, I had been given a clean bill of health. So no one knew. The sinking pit in my stomach kept growing during the last two blocks to the doctor's.

When I walked in, I was immediately ushered back. No waiting. You know it's a bad sign when they don't even ask for your copay first. I stared blankly at the wall as I waited for my primary care physician. A short while later, she walked in, solemn faced, and gave me the news. My tumor markers had doubled once in two weeks, and then doubled again during the following two weeks. This indicated that "something" in my body was spinning out of control. I sat there dumbfounded.

First, my doctor told me to cancel work for the rest of the day. I needed to get a CT scan, an MRI, and a bone scan. She had already made the appointments for me because she was well acquainted with my treatment facilities and medical teams. And she had already been on the phone with my oncologist and surgeon. They were looped into the situation and would be handling my case as it moved forward. Alone, I headed for my CT scan.

I called my parents on the way. They were not at home, so I left a message on their machine. This would blindside them. Then I called my office and requested the rest of the day off due to an "emergency." My manager was understanding, thank goodness, and didn't ask me to explain.

The next three days were a blur. I went through more tests than I wish to remember. I talked several times a day to my parents, who drove in from some distance away to endure the tests and doctors' appointments with me. Each appointment brought more bad news. When we got the confirmation twenty-four hours later that my cancer had indeed returned, I sat on my futon and, while I still had the emotional strength to do it, I started paging through my address book and then called my friends. All were shocked. I drove over to Donna's house to give her and her husband the news. It happened to be their second anniversary. I was originally diagnosed three weeks after their wedding. Donna had joked that her anniversary was the harbinger of bad news from me, but last year I'd happily sent a celebratory card reporting no news other than my joy for their continued happiness. Not this year.

Later, about two months into chemotherapy for the cancer that had now spread to my bones, liver, and lungs, I tried to make sense of the whole thing. I had never been one to research breast cancer. I'd avoided the statistics and the predictions. I figured that I was already the rarity for being diagnosed so young—so what did this research have to do with me?

But one morning, as I was struggling at work, watching the snow fall in the parking lot, and wishing that I was outside making snow angels instead of working part time and trying to figure out what to do with my life, I got an unquenchable thirst to find out "why." So I went to a local bookstore over lunch.

I picked up *Dr. Susan Love's Breast Book*, also known as the "breast cancer bible," and began to read. This was quite possibly the first piece of literature I'd ever picked up about breast cancer—I had gladly given my original gifted copy to someone else years before. Now I went right to the chapter on recurrence. It described the symptoms and where the cancer traditionally metastasized. Usually when it goes to the bones (the first place), you feel back pain and general achiness. (That started around June 2000.) The cancer usually goes to the lungs next, which is evident by the wheezing sound that comes with each breath taken. I had thought I was just winded from carrying those laptops around and working out obsessively. Guess I was wrong! When it gets to the liver, you can't tell so much by outward symptoms; the blood counts give you this news. For the first time during my cancer ordeal, I felt better. I was the textbook case of recurrence. But that didn't prepare me for what I read next.

If the cancer is caught when it reaches the bones initially, the ongoing prognosis and treatment options are good. However, if the cancer goes undetected until it reaches the lungs and liver, only 5 percent of patients live a year and 2 percent live two years following the diagnosis. WHAT? Let me re-read that. Two percent make it for two years. Where's the paragraph after that?

There wasn't one.

I did some quick math. I was twenty-six. I was diagnosed a second time in October 2000. It was December now, so according to the breast cancer bible, I would be, at best, dead in twenty-two months at the age of twenty-eight.

As I read Dr. Love's "bible," tears welled up in my eyes. I felt faint. I'd never had "that" discussion with my doctors before: the "How long do I have, Doc?" discussion. No wonder they had been so adamant about starting treatment immediately. No wonder they had breathed a sigh of relief when they could tell from the MRI that the cancer had not spread to my brain. (The breast cancer bible would not even discuss prognosis for a patient whose metastasis had reached the brain.) No wonder, since my mother, father, brother, and friends had done the research before I had, they cried when they called me. According to this, I had twenty-two months left to live—if I was in the top 2 percent, that is.

I took the rest of the day off from work. I mean, with twenty-two months left to live, who wants to create a training brochure? I went home and cried again. And again. And again. I had no one to call to tell about my new knowledge. From my friends' initial responses, I figured they already knew. The only stories they had shared with me were "miracle" stories; stories of the unexplained healing of cancer patients. Now I understood why. I had twenty-two months left to live, and the clock was ticking.

Jana once explained what it feels like to be diagnosed with cancer so young. We have a "sense of urgency" when it comes to our accomplishments and goals. Life seems more precious. You "stop to smell the roses"—although, after all my crying, my nose felt too stuffy to smell much of anything. I'd never made a "Things to Do Before I Die" list, but I didn't want to start now because doing so would acknowledge the inevitability of death that now loomed closer than ever. Was I ready to die? Had I done what I needed to do on earth? Was I ready to meet my maker?

That question "Am I ready to die?" is what got me through the next couple of months. It took quite a bit of time for me to answer in a way I was comfortable with. In trying to answer the question, I felt freer to live. It was a growing process as I realized that I'd had a good life here on earth, but the image of the ever-after was even more comforting.

I can relate to people who, during times of suffering, just wish to be done with it all. I think what waits for me is pain-free, guilt-free, animosity-free, and judgment-free, with an unlimited supply of Yankee Candles and diet Dr. Pepper.

I learned to be more laid back. I mean, what is the worst that can happen with twenty-two months left to live? Who would want to waste time accusing someone of rumored hatefulness if there are only twenty-two months left? Who would insist that the events of the day hinge on the global roll-out of a cell phone application when there are only twenty-two months left to live? Conversely, who would miss a family event, no matter how far away? Or the wedding of a close friend? It became a great life simplifier.

And when I reached November 2002—more than twenty-two months later—I felt as though I were living on "grace time."

If I had always lived as though I had twenty-two months left to live, I would have told more people that I loved them during my first twenty-six years. I would have skinned my knees more, put that trip to Africa on my credit card, and spent less time at work and more time at the BBQ grill at a friend's house.

I began living like that when I learned I had only twenty-two more months to live. You dream a bit more, achieve a bit more, let less bother you, worry about time less, and give more hugs. You laugh a lot more, eat more ice cream, travel more, worry less, moisturize more, dance more, exercise less, call friends more, and develop more meaning in your life.

With twenty-two months to live, I forgave the people who had hurt me, and I forgot about hurtful situations more quickly. With twenty-two months left, I wanted those people to be a part of my life. I started subscribing to *Real Simple* magazine and I discontinued my *Cosmo* subscription (although I still bought it at the newsstand each month!). I tried to eat healthier food and follow my "cancer diet" exactly as the book prescribed. But when I wanted dessert for dinner, I ate it. I mean, with twenty-two months left to live, who cares if they open me up and find my liver filled with French silk pie? I learned to cry when I felt sad. I learned to ask for help. I think in opening my heart to the infinite sadness of having only twenty-two months to live, I, in turn, learned to love unconditionally, shamelessly, and without regard to what stipulations others may have placed on me. I learned to practice agape love.

It's a shame that it took me having twenty-two months to live to learn how.

In the twenty-two months after my recurrence, I discovered a strength of heart and a depth of will I did not know I had. I learned to live without fear of future diagnoses and to move forward among friends with hope and love. Learning to live through those twenty-two months prepared me for month twenty-three and beyond.

Jana

There are 1,826 days in five years. In the cancer world, five years is a big deal. If you survive for five years after being diagnosed, the prognosis typically improves and the chance for a recurrence or metastasis generally decreases. At least that is what the statistics say. Others say that once the five-year mark is reached, you are in "remission" and are "cancer free."

I was surprised to learn that there is a controversy in the cancer world about when the clock starts counting those 1,826 days. Is it the day you discovered your lump, whether through a BSE or a mammogram, even though it was not yet confirmed to be cancer? Is it the day you were diagnosed and told you had cancer? Does the clock begin after your treatment ends? For breast cancer, is it five years after your mastectomy (if you had one), or five years after you finished radiation (if you had that), or is it five years after you started or ended chemotherapy (if you had chemo)? The controversy boggles my mind.

Even more mind-boggling to me is the controversy about when you are considered "cured" or in "remission." Although some cancers are curable, breast cancer is not. Though hundreds of thousands of women who are diagnosed continue to live long, fully productive lives, they still technically have breast cancer. Researchers continue to work to find a cure, but until one is found, the question "Can it happen to me again?" will always, always, always, linger in the back of my mind.

My personal opinion on the "five-year anniversary date" controversy is this: The day I was told I had breast cancer is the day my life turned upside down. Even though I already knew I had a lump, I did not know for certain that it was cancer. And, even though I had to have a mastectomy, the surgery date was not the day my life took a 180-degree turn. The day I was told I had cancer was the day that changed the rest of my life. Therefore, my clock started that day. I figure that although all of those other events are worthy of being considered milestones, I just don't consider them part of my official "1,826-day calendar."

Prognostic factors are things that doctors look at when a breast cancer diagnosis is made. Factors such as tumor size, location, and whether or not lymph nodes are involved result in the "staging" of the cancer. There are Stages I through IV. Stage I has the best prognosis and Stage IV the worst. Another prognostic factor is the tumor's pathology. For example, doctors try to determine whether or not the tumor is reactive to the female hormones estrogen and progesterone (also called ER and/or PR positive). There is also a test called HER2 receptor status. A tumor can have all, some, or none of these factors. Those that are ER/PR positive and HER2 negative typically are considered favorable prognostic factors. Age is also a factor. The younger you are when you are diagnosed, the more aggressive the cancer usually is. This is not a good prognostic factor.

In my case, the only prognostic factor I had against me was my age. I was Stage I when diagnosed, and my lymph nodes were negative. My tumor was HER2 negative and ER/PR positive. With these factors, I should not have to worry about whether or not the cancer could happen to me again. But even after a mastectomy, prophylactic chemotherapy, and my good prognosis, I knew that breast cancer could happen again. I tried to remember that factors were in my favor against recurrence whenever the question entered my thoughts.

As a newlywed, I quickly filled my life with work, the usual activities of daily living, and being a wife. I enjoyed having my life back on track. My hair had grown back, I had returned to work, I had regained energy, and my vasculitis reaction to chemo had finally been resolved. Chris and I celebrated my "one year since being diagnosed with breast cancer" milestone, and our married life became more settled and calming. I began to look forward to our first wedding anniversary and to the continued partnership with Chris that our marriage provided.

Of course, there were stressful times during the newlywed year. The days leading up to the frequent medical check-ups. The blood tests and the scans. These were followed by a huge sigh of collective relief after the results came back as "negative" or "no change." With each good news report, Chris and I began to plan more for our long-term future. Although the lingering question of whether or not the cancer would come back was always with us, we gained confidence that the cancer saga was behind us—after all, my prognosis was good!

About 487 days into the pursuit of my magical five-year milestone, I felt severe pain in my chest, neck, and upper back. I attributed it to my being a "road warrior." When I traveled, I carried my laptop computer inside a less-than-ergonomic backpack. Also, it was October, National Breast Cancer Awareness Month, and I had lifted several heavy boxes loaded with pink-ribbon tee shirts and breast cancer awareness materials to set up at information tables during my weekends.

However, the pain finally became so unrelenting that I went to see my primary care physician. He prescribed some anti-inflammatory medicine and a muscle relaxant. But the medications didn't help. In fact, my pain worsened. I went back, and this time he prescribed a mild narcotic to go along with the other medications. I did not like taking prescription drugs, but I was desperate to alleviate the pain.

I was beginning to worry. Could I be experiencing bone metastasis pain? I was concerned enough to ask my doctor whether he "wanted to take a chest x-ray, to see if everything is okay." He emphatically replied, "There is no way that this could be related to your breast cancer." Because I wanted to believe him, and because I was too busy to pursue my fear, I decided to trust my doctor for the time being.

The pain continued in November. Again, I asked for an x-ray. I felt as if I had a broken bone and was also suffering severe muscle tension.

I was constantly thinking that it could be cancer again. Then I'd tell myself I was simply scared. After all, I was barely seventeen months out of my original diagnosis, and I had just celebrated my first wedding anniversary. I did not have time for breast cancer again!

During a mid-December business trip to Chicago, I was rushing to O'Hare to catch my flight home. It was snowing and bitterly cold. There was murky slush in the gutters and on the sidewalks, and as I stepped out of the shuttle van, I slipped on some slush that had turned to ice. I caught myself from falling by grabbing the roof of the van with one hand. Pain seared my body. It felt as if a rib spreader had opened my chest and separated my sternum from my ribs. I got hot and clammy and almost vomited. Sheer will and adrenaline carried me and my suitcase into the terminal, where I collapsed. I sat smack down against a wall under some flight monitors. At this moment, I had a strong feeling the cancer had spread. I also knew I had to get home, but I could not move. Giant tears welled up in my eyes and poured down my cheeks.

There were lots of things wrong with this picture. First, I am so vigilant about germs in public places that I would never sit on the floor of an airport, let alone a dirty, slushy, and muddy floor like the one at O'Hare that day. Second, I rarely cry in public. Third, I am a strong woman, and I have a sense of invincibility. But there I was, sitting on the floor like a crumpled, broken puppet, and the only thing I was able to do was call Chris and hope his strength could get me through. I told him that I couldn't make the flight home because I couldn't move and that I had cancer again.

One of the best things about Chris is the calming effect he has on me. He reminded me that I was strong. I could do this. He reminded me that the flight was not a long one and that he would meet me at the airport upon my return. And, perhaps most important, he said a prayer all the way through the static of our cell phone connection. He asked God to give me the strength and courage to make it home. And I did.

The next day, I went to my oncologist's office rather than my primary care physician's office. The pain was at its most severe, and I could barely even move my neck. Each movement of my sternum, even something as small as breathing, hurt. A bone scan was ordered. When the bone scan technician told me the radiologist wanted "a couple more views and an x-ray," I knew my worst fear was being realized: I have cancer again, and it has spread to my bones.

The scans showed several "hot spots" (areas of cancer) in my sternum and on my hip bone, so a bone biopsy was ordered for my sternum. It was just a few days before Christmas.

The day after my bone biopsy, my oncologist called. I was on my lunch hour, and I was talking on my cell phone while waiting at a red light. She told me that it was indeed cancer; I would need to make an appointment to see her as soon as possible to develop a treatment plan.

I was near my office, so I drove there and parked my car. But I couldn't go in to work. Instead, I called Chris and began to cry. I couldn't speak. He knew exactly what was wrong. I did not have to tell him. After composing myself and convincing him I was "safe" to drive, we decided to meet at home as soon as possible. I called my boss and told her that I had a medical emergency and would not be back that afternoon, and then I drove home. It was much like being diagnosed the first time: After our tears had dried and we had said a long prayer, we made phone calls and set prayer chains in motion.

Then followed a whirlwind of medical tests, scans, and doctors' appointments. It was just like the first time I was diagnosed. The only difference was that instead of a tumor in my breast, I had bone "mets" (the lingo for metastasis).

I saw my medical oncologist and radiation oncologist. The oncologists recommended radiation treatment to my sternum to kill the cancer and alleviate my severe pain. When a treatment is given to resolve pain, it is considered a palliative, not a curative treatment. I was concerned when my radiation oncologist told me that the treatment would not kill all the cancer cells in my sternum. Since there was also a hot spot on my hip bone, it was likely that there were cancer cells in other areas of my bones that had not shown up yet. He did say that surviving cancer cells in my sternum would become disabled; therefore I would not have to worry that cancer would spread from my sternum. He was very clear, however, that radiation was not a cure.

I had never had radiation and didn't know what to expect. First, I was measured, scanned, and x-rayed. This took well over an hour. The results were used to create a technical radiation treatment plan that mapped out how deeply the electrons could penetrate into bone but not go past into the vital organs, such as my lungs and heart, that lay beneath my breast bone.

When my custom treatment plan had been developed, a special plastic-and-lead plate was made to place in the radiation machine. It looked like something I had made in metal shop class in eighth grade. In the middle there was a hole shaped like the outline of my sternum; this was called the radiation portal. The radiation beam would go through the portal to the location that had been precisely targeted.

I started treatment a few days before the 2000 New Year, so as I said good-bye to the twentieth century and hello to the new millennium, I was glowing with radiation! I required fifteen treatments (I called them "zaps"). After my tenth zap, I was exhausted. I later learned that the dose of radiation I was receiving was a concentrated high dose, and because blood cells are made in the bones (in the sternum in particular), the radiation was killing healthy cells as well as cancer cells. No wonder I was fatigued.

After the long radiation preparation appointment, I was surprised when the actual zap took only a few minutes. In fact, it took longer to go to the clinic, undress, put on a too-large medical gown, and then dress again than it did to get the zap. And although it was inconvenient to go in for my zap every weekday, patients who had to go for six or more weeks of radiation had to endure far more inconvenience than I did. I really couldn't complain.

Fortunately, I was able to continue working during my treatments. Typically, I would work half a day in the office and half a day at home. Thank goodness for laptop computers, the Internet, and a flexible employer! With the exception of the fatigue and a bright red "sunburn" shaped like a T-bone steak on my chest, the process was uneventful. The skin redness was caused by the radiation. After my treatments ended, the skin peeled, and I had a tanned area on my chest for several months.

After five radiation treatments, my pain lessened considerably. This gave me a glimmer of hope—it meant the cancer cells were being eradicated. The treatment was working.

When my radiation treatments ended, my medical oncologist recommended two treatments that would become either lifelong or would last until my cancer spread elsewhere. My new treatments were a shocking reality.

The first option included either a total surgical hysterectomy or a chemical hysterectomy, the latter with a drug called Zoladex. Whichever treatment I chose would shut down my ovaries (the majority of estrogen and progesterone is produced in the ovaries). This treatment was advised because my tumor was reactive to the female hormones. The thought was that by decreasing the amount of these hormones in my body, any remaining cancer cells would starve.

I opted for the chemical hysterectomy with Zoladex, primarily because it would be easier than a surgical hysterectomy, and less risky, too. Also, the effects are reversible. That meant I could still have children if I stopped the injections.

The Zoladex injection itself was very painful. The needle was huge; it pierced my abdomen and deposited a pellet of medication that would last for three months. Thank goodness I only had to get this injection four times a year. Taking Zoladex caused full-blown menopause—and I was only twenty-nine years old!

Because I can't take hormone replacement therapy for my premature menopause, I am concerned that, over the long term, the premature menopause may increase my risk for heart disease and osteoporosis. However, I figure that by the time I'm old enough to worry about those things, medical treatments will have improved. I try not to worry about it now.

The second treatment my doctors recommended was a drug called Aredia, a bisphosphonate that strengthens bones. I was at high risk for breaking a bone as a result of the bone mets and the menopause. As with the Zoladex, I must continue on this plan until one of two things happens: Either I get worse because the cancer spreads to an organ, or I die.

Aredia was administered as an infusion, so I had to get an IV every month. With my initial chemotherapy, the fragile veins in my right hand were used. However, the toxicity of the chemo treatments had wreaked havoc on those veins; after my first infusion of Aredia, I had a painful reaction whereby my veins, hand, and arm turned red and became swollen and painful. As a result, I was advised to have a permanent Port-a-Cath inserted (the procedure is done on an outpatient basis). The port was implanted just below my right collar bone and then secured to my chest muscle. The tubing went directly into my heart. This type of port is called a "central line" for my vein. The port will be in my body for the rest of my life unless I get an infection or the device occludes (gets blocked) and stops working.

I was pleased when my thoughtful surgeon told me she had placed the port in such a way that I can still wear a bathing suit. When my body was thin, there was a visible "bump" under my skin where the port was. Since then, I have gained weight and it is virtually hidden in my fat tissue.

Before I started the Zoladex and the Aredia treatments, and after my radiation treatment ended, I pursued a second opinion at M. D. Anderson Cancer Center (MDA) in Houston, Texas.

Chris, my stepmom, and I traveled to this world-renowned cancer center and stayed for a full week. Here I had more medical and blood tests, saw several oncologists and residents in training to be oncologists, and had my medical reports reviewed and scrutinized.

The experience was humbling. At check-in, I was one of hundreds of other patients, most of them accompanied by friends or family members, who were waiting to register. The distressing reality is that we all had one thing in common: cancer.

I was surprised that one of my appointments for a CT scan occurred as late as 9:00 P.M.! This is because the hospital performed tests that late in the day in order to accommodate the large number of patients who needed them.

The MDA oncologists agreed to the regimen prescribed at home. This meant that the treatments I was having were the best ones for me and that I could feel secure in that knowledge as I proceeded.

By 2003, I reached my 1,826th day, a time of celebration and reflection. Because I'd continued my treatment for the bone metastasis, I did not technically have a clean bill of health. However, my CT and bone scans taken shortly after my five-year anniversary showed "no change," which was good news.

On day 1,827, I decided that it was "safe" to focus on my future. It was also time to consider seriously a prophylactic mastectomy with double reconstruction: the same procedure that Jen had undergone.

Technically, the surgery is elective; however, it was recommended for me because it would reduce by more than 90 percent my chances of developing breast cancer in my other breast.

In addition, I would no longer have a "fake boob." I'd have not only breast symmetry but also a heightened sense of self-esteem concerning my self-image and my body image.

For personal reasons, I opted for a double reconstruction with implants rather than the TRAM flap surgery that Patti and Kim had undergone. After bilateral mastectomies, the cosmetic results are typically more symmetrical if implants are used. Also, I had watched a TRAM flap surgery on *Discovery Health*, so I knew how the procedure was done; the idea that abdominal fat and muscle would be tunneled through my torso and then "pasted" to my chest haunted me.

The major choice I had to make about implants was between saline or silicone. The FDA removed silicone implants from the market when a possible link was discovered between leaking silicone and autoimmune dysfunction. However, I could still get a silicone implant if I entered a program in which I registered with the FDA and agreed to be followed for several years. Although a silicone implant is thought to feel and look more like a natural breast, I didn't want to risk leakage, so I chose saline. It would still be a big improvement over my fake boob and "uni-breast."

My surgery was scheduled for November 2003 and would be performed by a plastic surgeon and a breast surgeon. I felt there was a strong chance that breast cancer, or at least a precancerous condition called ductal carcinoma in situ (DCIS), might be found in the "healthy" breast. I had a gut feeling that something was not "right" again, and I was prepared to hear bad news.

When I awoke from my surgery, Chris was sitting on my hospital bed, holding my hand. His eyes held a deep sorrow as he told me the doctors had found more cancer. I said, "I know." I was not surprised until he told me that it was not in my healthy breast but in the chest-wall muscle behind my first mastectomy. I believe it was divine intervention that when my plastic surgeon incised my muscle to insert my tissue expander, the incision was at exactly the spot where the cancer was hiding. If I had not undergone the reconstruction surgery, the breast cancer may not have been found until it was too late.

My plastic surgeon removed the suspicious lump and had it analyzed. When it proved to be cancer, my breast surgeon placed permanent metal clips where the cancer was found so that she could locate the spot after surgery. She also removed some additional muscle in hopes of getting all the cancer cells. I will never know whether this cancer was a new growth or had lain hidden since my original diagnosis five and a half years earlier. In the end, it really didn't matter because cancer already had spread to my bones. However, with the chest-wall involvement, I now faced more radiation treatments.

Prior to implant surgery, I had to go through a process of tissue expansion with expanders. In chapter 6, Jen explained how that works. I will add only that the pain of adding saline solution to my expanders was so intolerable that it literally pinned me to the exam table during each "fill-up," as I called this step. I felt an intense tightness on my chest wall, and my chest muscles began to go into spasm. Next, my back muscles went into spasm.

The next week, the pain was even more intense, but I was a lady on a mission, and with gritted teeth, I let the doctor put in 100 cubic centimeters of saline. The purpose of my rapid fill-up was completely self-driven. I could not begin radiation until my expanders were at capacity, and I wanted to start radiation as quickly as possible. So I pushed myself. My plastic surgeon said I could do 50 cubic centimeters every other week, but in my mind, I didn't have time to waste. In four sessions, I reached 450 cubic centimeters in each tissue expander. But I paid a price. Pain kept me in bed for two full days. Chris helped me maintain an around-the-clock pain pill regimen, but it was only partially successful.

I went back to my radiation oncologist with a heavy heart. I knew radiation would be longer than the fifteen-day treatment on my sternum. This time, thirty-three zaps were prescribed, to be administered over six weeks.

Unlike before, I decided to go on short-term disability and spend time to recover. This was the right decision for me because radiation fatigue hit much harder this time. Also, I needed time to process the fact that this was my second recurrence. I had to work through a barrage of emotions.

My medical oncologist recommended that I continue with Zoladex and Aredia and that I add the "next line" of hormonal therapy. While at MDA, I had learned about "next line" treatments. In short, if the disease progresses, or if a particular treatment is not successful, other drugs may be given. Each drug is considered a different "line." The only time I will not move to a different "line" of treatment is if the cancer spreads to one of my organs—my liver, lungs, or brain. If that happens, the only option will be chemotherapy.

In the years since my initial diagnosis, a new class of drugs, called aromatase inhibitors (AIs), had been introduced. AIs stop the production of estrogen from the adrenal glands and from muscle and fat tissues. One of these AIs is called Femara, and I was started on it. A few weeks later, I had a serious reaction. A severe rash erupted over my chest and abdomen. For five straight days, Chris and I visited different specialists; when we finally saw my immunologist, he said, "It could be anything." He prescribed high doses of Prednisone and antihistamines that fortunately stopped, or at least suppressed, the reaction. My medical oncologist decided not to start any other new drugs until after I had completed radiation.

When I was diagnosed with breast cancer at age twenty-seven, I felt certain I was going to kick cancer's butt. When my breast cancer spread to my bones eighteen months later, it occurred to me for the first time that breast cancer would probably kill me. But I thought that day was twenty or thirty years in the future, and to me, that would still be like kicking cancer's butt. Today, I am not certain I am going to kick cancer's butt, but I don't think it will kick mine. That's because I have accepted the fact that I am not in control of the disease. I am only in control of how I deal with it. So I will continue with the prescribed medical regimens. I will have the most positive attitude I can. And I will live each day as if it were my last—because it could be.

I want to have more good days than bad, but I appreciate and treasure all days. When I wake up in the morning, I don't ask myself, "Is it time to get up already?!" Instead, I think to myself, "I am being blessed to live another day! This is one more day I have to glorify God by trying to make a positive difference in someone else's life."

Because I have seen the reality that cancer can return, I feel that each day I live is like winning the lottery of life. I am alive and kicking, and while I am, I'm going to serve God and fulfill my purpose. This year, more than forty-one thousand women will die from breast cancer in the United States. I hope I am not one of them. But breast cancer has changed my life for the better, and I would not change that. The lessons I have learned and the wisdom I obtain every day are all part of the bittersweet reality of this disease.

Jen

The "R" word is the one most feared by cancer survivors. You give it your all when you are initially diagnosed, and then you play the waiting game. I attended a cancer support group comprised of women being treated for a variety of cancers, though mostly breast cancer. Some were experiencing recurrences, and seeing these otherwise normal women facing their mortality was almost more than I could handle.

When I read the chapter on recurrence in *Dr. Susan Love's Breast Book*, it made me panic. I knew there was no guarantee that the treatment I had gone through would cure me. But how would I know whether I was having a recurrence? Thankfully, I had found my breast tumor, but what should I look for now? I read through the list of symptoms: bone pain, headaches, changes in the breast or mastectomy site, chest pain, shortness of breath, changes in weight. The list went on and on.

The next day, I felt a pain in my back and arm. I knew I had to be imagining it because I had just read Dr. Love's book, but it scared me. For about a week, I was so focused on a recurrence and the thought of dying that I started getting depressed. Matt promptly took the book away from me and hid it in the basement. I mean no disrespect to Dr. Love. Her book is known as the breast cancer "gospel." I was just not mentally prepared to read the chapter on recurrence.

One of the best things I did to ease my fears of recurrence and dying was to borrow a series of cancer tapes. For a few weeks I put off listening to the tape on dying, but it turned out to be surprisingly beautiful. It stressed that dying is actually very peaceful. It is being born into this world that comes with a lot of pain and crying.

Somehow the tape brought peace to my heart. If I did not survive this disease, I knew I had given it my all. I would make sure that all those I loved knew that I loved them. And I would make sure things were right between God and me.

I decided to focus on living and taking chances. I would have no regrets whether I lived to a hundred or to thirty. I was sent here for a purpose: to raise my little boy and help other women who may follow in my footsteps. That's what I would do.

Getting to know Jana and Patti also marked a turning point in how I viewed recurrence. Before getting to know them, recurrence was a death sentence in my mind. The odds were minimal that either of them would face a recurrence after a Stage I diagnosis. They had both been very aggressive with their treatments and were living healthy, active lives.

Although you need early detection, aggressive treatment, and a positive attitude, you also need a pinch of good luck. It's hard to understand why they have had to endure so much. Sometimes I feel guilty that so far I seem to be doing well. When they chatted about their latest Zoladex injection or infusion treatment, my heart hurt for them. I didn't want them to have to sit through any more treatments. It also scared me, because it could happen to me at any time (although most re-currences happen during the first two to five years).

Being around Jana and Patti helped me understand that, although dealing with a recurrence sucks, life does go on. The resolve that these women shared was amazing. For them, treatment was an inconvenience, but it was only a small part of their lives. I can only hope to be half as graceful if cancer reenters my life.

Time has been a great healer for me. The further I am from my diagnosis, the less I think about the possibility of recur-rence. It's no longer part of every waking moment. I asked Lisa, a cancer friend I met at church, when I would stop obsessing over it. What she told me was so true. It would take baby steps, she said. First an hour would go by without my thinking about it, then half a day. Finally, an entire day would pass. When that actually happened, I realized that I was in a race that would be won not with a quick sprint but with a slow, steady pace.

Breast cancer is a part of my life. I know there is still a slim chance for a recurrence, but instead of worrying, I have chosen to embrace life and make the most of it. I am still Jennifer John-son, mother, wife, daughter, coworker, and friend. I will not live my life in fear of something over which I have no control. Let-ting go of the fear of death was the most liberating part of my ex-perience. In the end, it is a blessing to realize at such an early age how precious life is while I have still time to make the most of it.

Kim

Fear is a word that comes to mind when someone is diagnosed with the big "C." I feared both the unknown and the known, such as losing my hair. But the biggest fear by far is that of recurrence. There is no "cure" for breast cancer. There is neither rhyme nor reason as to who experiences a metastasis and who doesn't.

Patti and Jana both had early-stage cancers, and both underwent aggressive treatments. Why did their cancer come back? How would I know if mine came back? Would I recognize the symptoms or simply put them off? I didn't want to be paranoid, requesting a bone scan with every little pain, but I also didn't want to ignore something that could be a sign.

The other issue that concerned me about a recurrence was that my pathology report indicated that my tumor was triple negative. My tumor was estrogen-negative, progesterone-negative, and HER2 negative. This meant that I was not a good candidate for hormone therapy, such as Tamoxifen. It also meant that I was not eligible for Herceptin, a drug that can help women who are HER2 positive if they have a recurrence. As it did Jen, it haunted me that I could not give my body extra treatment. And for me, if my cancer does return, there are not any new drugs available for me. This is very frustrating, particularly when I hear about all the clinical trials, studies, and new drugs coming out—none of which would help me.

Patti's aggressive treatments were similar to mine the first time around. Besides Jana, I knew several other young women whose breast cancer had metastasized. Some of them didn't make it. This really freaked me out. On my second round of chemo, I remember sitting next to a woman in her early fifties. She had first been diagnosed eight years earlier, and now her cancer had metastasized to her bones, liver, lungs, and brain. Her prognosis was not good, but she was in good spirits. She said she had spoken to a woman who had been having treatments for ten years for metastasized cancer, and she was still around. This made me feel good for her, but at the same time, scared.

What if I go through all this and then it comes back?

The first year after my initial diagnosis, the fear of recurrence was always in the back of my mind. Every little ache or pain caused anxiety. I feared my lab results at every check-up. I was fearful of a suspicious bone scan. I was fearful of a suspicious mammogram. Simply, I was fearful of death. My doctor and I agreed on a ten-day rule: Pain that persisted longer than ten days should be checked out.

Four months after my final chemotherapy treatment, I experienced back pain. Immediately, I thought about Patti. After ten days of pain, my doctor agreed to schedule a bone scan. The scan came back clean, and my peace of mind was restored. (I've heard some women who have symptoms for only a day or two are tested and are at Stage IV.)

My oncologist didn't believe in the routine of tumor-marker tests every three months. He said that they often produce false positives and that there were other variables—such as stress—that could contribute to raised tumor markers. If my cancer should come back, by the time it showed up on a tumor marker test, I would already have other symptoms, he said. I wasn't too sure about his theory and I questioned him at length. Many other women had these tests, and I wanted them, too. In my search for answers, my doctor provided me with several medical journal articles. But, especially after questioning other doctors, I persisted. Ultimately, my doctor agreed to give me the blood tests along with my regular litany of other tests: chest x-ray, bone scan, and mammogram.

This oncologist moved away shortly after that, and my new oncologist regularly performs the tumor marker test. It shows that every doctor is different and that it is important to become educated and insist on doing what feels comfortable for you—I made sure I was a part of the medical team.

With each year that passes, the fear of recurrence lessens. Anxiety still overcomes me when I go for a check-up. Will my tests come back clear? Yet watching Jana and Patti deal with their recurrences has helped me realize that I cannot let fear overcome me. They showed such a zest for life. I was amazed by their spirit and courage. Although I angrily questioned why their cancer came back, I saw that they were not letting it get in their way. Eventually, I knew I shouldn't let it get in my way, either. If I lived every waking moment paralyzed by fear, I was not truly living.

Patti taught me that I had a precious gift—my life. Even though she had a recurrence and knew her prognosis wasn't good, she lived each day as a gift. I wanted to do the same.

Fear of recurrence did make me acknowledge the reality of death. I even became practical enough to write down my funeral requests so that Scott would know what I wanted.

Then I set about living. I don't think I'm going to die of breast cancer. I think I'm going to grow into a wise old woman who enjoys her golden years on a beach somewhere with the love of my life.

Worrying does not empty tomorrow of its troubles—it empties today of its strength.

AUTHOR UNKNOWN

If my cancer does come back, I'll deal with it. And I'll fight as hard as I fought my first battle. Meanwhile, I'll continue to live each day as a gift from God.

CHAPTER EIGHT

Relationships and Intimacy

— Nordie's Café —
January 2003

F riends and family, the birds and the bees, body image—that's practically all we talk about, right?" said Kim. "I mean where would late twenties/early thirtysomething girls be, without conversations about religion, friends, work, sex, and breasts?"

We wanted to write a chapter about relationships and intimacy. It was easy to talk about these things at our table, where we could parallel our relationship foibles with stories from friends or our favorite television shows. But the move from pop culture to personal wasn't that easy. We'd often imagined ourselves as the *Sex and the City* girls—where the excitement or hurt came in half-hour doses, complete with a soft couch and a sugary snack. It slowly dawned on us that although the show's characters experienced doubts and fears about relationships, when those were translated from the small screen to our own lives, the concerns were our own, too. And how we chose to grapple with them was a fundamental expression of who we were and how we decided to live with breast cancer.

We had experienced severe trauma to our young bodies. Patti joked, "At what point in dating do you tell the guy,

'Yeah, these aren't real, and by the way, I have Stage IV breast cancer'?"

We moved from the slightly racy to the profound in minutes—from the enjoyment of sex to fundamental changes in relationships—and wrote our ideas in this chapter. Maybe we did act a bit like the *Sex and the City* characters of Carrie (Patti), Miranda (Jana), Charlotte (Jen), and Samantha (Kim) when we gathered around the table with our lipstick-stained glasses and bantered about why men like us or not, about what everyone thinks about breasts. But then, this was our own show. We hope it will inspire others to relate to us and begin their own conversations.

Patti

When I heard that my tumor markers had come back elevated for the second time in a month, I knew my cancer had returned. I went to church and prayed, "I just really, really, really need a sign. I need a sign to know that this isn't going to be it for me."

Everything had indicated that the cancer was not coming back. So why was it back? I didn't have the same instinct to fight as I did during my first bout. This time I really felt as if I were going to die. I called my brother in Africa. He was almost finished with his Peace Corps tour. I called the Peace Corps office and told them I wanted him to come home. I thought, "If it can come back and multiply and multiply and multiply this much in the course of a month, then think about what it's going to take to get me through this."

I went to bed that night knowing that I'd get my CT scan results in the next couple of days. Those would tell me how "bad" the recurrence was. I prayed again the same "I need a sign" prayer. I didn't sleep well because how can you sleep well when you have been told that your cancer has returned and you are waiting on CT scan results to see how "bad" it is?

I woke up the next morning at six o'clock. It was rainy and overcast. I did not want to get up, so I willed myself back to sleep. Eight o'clock came, more rain, and still I did not feel ready to face the day. I decided to stay in bed a bit longer. Ten o'clock rolled around, and I was awakened with a little sunbeam on my head. I felt as if someone were talking to me—and this is where it will get a little weird for some readers.

I was lying on my back, face up to the ceiling, when a "voice" in my head said something to me. Suddenly, I was wide awake. I asked the voice, "So are you telling me that this is not it for me?" It was almost as if I heard someone say, "Yep, it's not it. This time is going to be harder for you; there will be places of downtime that you have never experienced before, but if you are faithful and keep on task, you'll get through it." The conversation continued. I said, "You're telling me once again, God, that this isn't it for me?" "Yes, that's what I'm telling you. You're going to have to lean on me. You're going to have to lean on others. But you'll get through it." At that moment, the clouds and rain returned.

I got out of bed, incredulous about what had just happened, and walked into the kitchen. My mother and grandmother were standing there. The only words out of my mouth were, "I get to stay." My mother and grandmother didn't understand. I repeated myself and told them the entire story. My mother started crying. My grandmother didn't get it at first—but she is a woman with really strong faith. Once she got it, she thought it was cool. I called my brother in Africa and said, "If you want to finish out your last month with the Peace Corps, you can. I'm going to be fine. It's going to suck, it's going to be far harder than last time, I guarantee you that, but I know what the outcome is." My experience with my recurrence hinged on that moment. It was the start of a very personal relationship with God.

During my recurrence, my support circle was smaller, but it was more effective. I pinpointed relationships that were meaningful to me. This meant that I let fewer people in. I let someone in when I knew I could trust that person unconditionally, and when I was comfortable about saying, "This is what I need from you; let's get together and let's do something." I shared updates and musings with thirty close friends in a biweekly e-mail I called "Journal of a Cancer Survivor." In my support network I included coworkers, friends from Bible study groups, sorority sisters, and family members.

I kept in touch with Chris #2. He came up with the idea that I needed to list all the people with whom I routinely interact to determine whether or not they fell into my "water basin." After three pages of instant messaging conversation via our computers, including a detailed geological explanation, I finally got it. It goes something like this (prepare to split your sides laughing): "You see, there is the continent of Patti [these were his real words]. Say, for instance, you are the Mississippi. There are bodies of water that flow into the Mississippi." "Like tributaries?" I questioned, pleased that I actually remembered that word. "Yes," he responded excitedly, probably glad that I was finally starting to get it. "The bodies of water that flow into your Mississippi are in your water basin. For instance, the water from the east side of Colorado flows into the Mississippi (meaning my water basin). But then there is the water that is on the western side of Colorado that doesn't flow into the Mississippi. This is still part of the U.S. of Patti." "Yes," I responded.

Chris was concerned that I had let too many people (I swear this is verbatim) "flow into my water basin . . . when they are really places of lesser consequence to the west of Colorado," the Utahs, as I'd taken to calling them by the end of the conversation.

After this explanation, he gave me the "water basin assignment." I was to figure out who on the continent of Patti flowed into my water basin—and who were the Utahs. I came up with an ominous list of people on my continent by combining my Christmas card list with a copy of my office directory—all to figure out who should, and who should not, flow into my water basin. For once (ha!), Chris was right—I realized that I had been spending too much energy keeping in touch with the Utahs.

The wedding of a good friend confirmed the water basin message even further. After the wedding, I was sitting with a group of people who were gossiping about the bride. I thought, "This is so hurtful and hateful, take me out of the loop." Why? I have a limited time on earth. Do I want to spend it gossiping about a friend on her wedding day? Or do I want to work to maintain a relationship with that friend?

During the second round of chemo, I became more comfortable about saying, "Hey, you're not a value-added to my life, see ya." I would have had a problem with that a long time ago. But right now, I reasoned, "I've got a lot on my plate and I'm busy adding meaningful things—you can either be a part of that meaning or not."

Dione and Donna were constant fixtures at my chemotherapy sessions. I also involved my family a lot more during the recurrence. At times, it was frustrating because I'm independent. During my first treatment, when I was sick during chemo, or if I passed out from dehydration, I'd get friends to drive me rather than call my parents for support. But my mom and dad were always there.

What amazed me was their sensitivity to my need for independence and their willingness to help when I did call or when they saw that I needed them. One weekend when I had painful spasms in my back, I called my mom and she drove up to be with me. After my first round of chemo, I gave thanks for my first meal, mashed potatoes, and my hero, Daddy, who brought them to me. When a new chemo regimen had unusually bad side effects, my dad brought cookies, which seemed to help alleviate the chemo side effects. He began promoting himself as a future Nobel Prize winner. By his reckoning, the chemo gets the cancer and Bob's Cookies cure any number of odd chemotherapy-induced side effects. All we had to do was have the oncologist write it up in a medical journal and buy plane tickets to Sweden for the ceremony. Well, he may never win the real Nobel Prize, but, as with any little girl, he remained my hero for saving the day once again. Knowing that my mom and dad were always there gave me immense emotional support. Throughout the treatment, they inspired me daily by the way they lived their lives, showing that problems can be solved through prayer, laughter, and hard work.

When my brother returned from Africa, people said that I began to look much better. I believe it is because he was here to joke with me and remind me that I am a bit anal-retentive, which also made me laugh. He was by far the light of my life. Without him keeping me up nights laughing by doing his impression of the rock band Oasis in my blonde wig, the first few months of round two would have been unbearable.

My second round of chemo treatment took longer, so I was able to invite more of my friends into the infusion room. This gave my friends and family a sense of being included in the healing process.

Although I loved the influx of cards that came right after my original diagnosis, the ones that came during months eight, nine, and on were especially meaningful. People like me want to get back to life as normal, so there's nothing like having a little something in my mailbox besides bills to remind me that someone special from far away is thinking of me.

As for dating relationships and thoughts of marriage—that was tough. After my original diagnosis and during my recurrence, I had my doubts about both. What I can say is this: When I had more energy, I pursued dating and boy relationships more seriously. But during periods of low energy, or when I gave serious thought to the fact that I could die in the near future, I pursued relationships out of a passion for love, joy, and friendship rather than a desire for intimacy. Regarding marriage, I went to lunch one day with my new "chemo friend," Jana. She told me how her husband married her the month after she finished chemotherapy, and although she had no fingernails, he took her on a honeymoon. I left lunch happy because I like making new friends. However, later I thought, "Wow, how great that she has a husband who loves her enough to take her for the two to fifty years that he might have with her."

Then it struck me, as I was driving back to work: I didn't think I deserved that. Somewhere in the past two years, I had equated marriage to a selling job. "I have a lot to offer you, so you should want to spend the rest of your life with me." But as cancer invaded my life, I felt my best selling points were slipping away. I have only one real breast, I can't carry or bear children, and the latest kicker: I might not even make it to our one-year anniversary. Why would anyone want to take that chance? I was (and I mean *was*) very unhappy about having to explain to a future spouse that I might die at any time.

In my mind, all that outweighed the nice, outstanding things I could bring to a marriage. Never mind that I had friends and family who truly valued me for all that I offered. Emotions don't always agree with solid logic. My marriage "realization" drove me into hiding under my covers (sweating menopause-profusely) for almost a month. Sometimes I just worked, came home, went to bed, and cried. Then, one day, spring came (literally and figuratively), and life seemed a little sunnier.

During the recurrence, I had a "no dating while having cancer" policy for a while. Later, I went out on a date every now and again and allowed myself to have crushes. However, it was my relationship with Chris #2 and our "best-friend-hood" that was a constant. As life got more difficult and I had less dating energy, I think I progressed from loving Chris to having a warm fuzzy feeling when we got together.

One unexpected set of relationships that flourished in my life were those between me and my coauthors, Jana, Jennifer, and Kim. Each of us had looked for breast cancer support groups, but found that often issues discussed at those groups weren't issues on the top of our list. For us, it was not "How do I make out a living will?" It was "Can I have kids some day?" "How should I argue for my promotion?" "Do I lose all my hair? Hmmm, I should tell my husband that." The weekly dose of laughter, comfort, and camaraderie was unmatched.

Listening to Jen, Jana, and Kim helped me come to terms with my fears about dating and romantic relationships.

At the end of the day, like a lot of things, it came down to knowing who I was and where I was. This, of course, made dating tricky. One weekend, I relished the attention and affection Chris #2 gave me on a float trip and thought about what our future would be like together. Another weekend, I would take safe haven in the companionship of Dione and Donna because I knew that my energy or psychology wasn't ready for dealing with the unknowns of a dating relationship.

The balance of all this was that I grew in faith, and was blessed with the support of family and close friends. Knowing they were there for me helped me retain my freedom to live fully despite the cancer.

Jana

After I was diagnosed with breast cancer, all my relationships seemed to change. My relationships with my fiancé, parents, sister, other family members, health care providers, friends, coworkers, and even strangers—all changed! I am not sure whether this was because of the way I interacted with others or whether it was because of the way others interacted with me. Probably a little bit of both.

Let me start with Chris. I was most concerned with how he would react to the physical changes caused by my cancer treatments. He was my fiancé and future husband, so what would he think of my missing breast and my shiny bald head? Would he be physically attracted to me any more? How would the physical changes caused by surgery and chemotherapy affect our love life and our ability to be intimate? Before I had cancer, I had a petite frame, complemented by size 36C breasts, and although I was not in great shape, I was healthy and wore size 6 jeans. I had flippy, fun hair. I felt attractive and I was loaded with confidence.

In addition to the outward physical changes, I wondered whether Chris would become bored with me when the extreme fatigue caused by chemotherapy set in. What if I was no longer "fun"? What if I was unable to maintain the "Energizer Bunny" pace of my precancer life, which was filled with excitement, travel, and spontaneity? Now I was facing a much slower pace and lifestyle. Sure, I knew that our relationship was more than these superficial things. But weren't these the initial things that had attracted Chris to me?

I was also worried that Chris's perception of our once pure, simple, and exciting future was now "tainted" with the reality that life could (and, at the moment, was) causing more pain than happiness. And I could—gasp—die! Before the cancer spread to my bones, we never really addressed the reality that I could die. In those "early years" of our marriage, I didn't think I would die from this disease. But what about the future, and having a family, and work, and the unknown?!?

Fortunately, Chris was always supportive and followed my lead in how to react to my physical and emotional changes. In fact, I believe that our relationship became stronger. We were building the foundation of our life together on solid rock—not on sand. If we could withstand cancer, and we were not even married yet, we thought we could handle anything marriage could bring! This feeling of invincibility was somewhat naïve, yet empowering, and it helped both of us through the ordeal.

"Intimacy" was another issue altogether. I believe there are two main aspects of intimacy: the emotional and the physical.

Chris made it clear from the day I was diagnosed that he was not marrying me for my breasts, he was marrying me for me; whatever it took for me to beat this disease, including the loss of a breast, was not an issue with him. Because of Chris's attitude, our physical relationship didn't change much.

Chris's acceptance of my new body was remarkable. He continued to make love to me as if I had two breasts. He didn't treat me as if I were "deformed," even though I often felt like that myself. He simply told me that my other breast would have to get extra attention, if necessary. And all the while I wondered whether this man was too good to be true. After all, I had heard horror stories of husbands telling their wives they were less of a woman without a breast or breasts. Although I like to think I would never become engaged to a man like that, I will admit that I had some feelings of insecurity, simply because of the emphasis of breasts on television, and even in the mailbox with each *Sports Illustrated* swimsuit issue and Victoria's Secret catalogue that arrived.

My relationship with my dad and stepmom was open and loving. In hindsight, my parents probably knew a lot more about me and my doings than I will ever realize, but they allowed me to explore, within limits, my personal need for independence and creativity. Nevertheless, it was unusual to be twenty-seven and living at home, as I was when first diagnosed.

Although I was working full time and making a nice living, because I traveled nearly every weekday and was home only on weekends, living with my parents meant I didn't have to worry about maintaining an apartment I would rarely live in.

I now believe I was "still" living at home for a reason—I needed to be there when I was diagnosed with breast cancer.

Even though I went on disability leave from work and maintained a salary and benefits, I enjoyed the company of my family. Had I already been married, things would have been different. But, as my circumstances were, family support was what I needed. And I think my parents needed it, too. They needed to see me each day as I had my highs and lows. They needed to see that even though the chemotherapy beat me down, I was okay. At the same time, it was very challenging to be in limbo between living at home, getting married, and being sick.

My then future in-laws were always very supportive of Chris and me. They lived several hours away, so they were removed from my daily battle with cancer. I am thankful that they did not have to see the day-to-day pain that Chris had to see me go through. When I was first diagnosed, I worried that my in-laws would be upset that I was putting their son through such a difficult experience at a time when we were celebrating our engagement. If they felt that way, they never let it show. Chris's parents were as unconditionally loving and supportive as if I were their own daughter. They have always welcomed and supported me and are remarkable people. Chris didn't fall far from the tree.

In the months following my "D-Day," my relationship with my sister, Angi, blossomed. Although she is only three years older than I am, we were not close while growing up and we lived in different cities from the time I was sixteen years old. From the day I was diagnosed, Angi became a key part of my support team, and she subsequently helped me through each recurrence. She has also been with me during my times of good health, and today I consider her one of my best friends. Our relationship is one of the few "good side effects" of having breast cancer.

It is true that you find out who your real friends are in the time of a crisis. Several friends whom I hadn't been close to for years came back into my life. It didn't matter that I had lost contact with them for a time. True friends are for life. On the flip side, some friends I thought would be there seemed to fall off the face of the earth after I was diagnosed. I think of them as my fair-weather friends.

My true friends fell into one of two categories: those who lived nearby and those who lived far away. Both were supportive in their own ways. Those who lived far away would e-mail, call, and send care packages and cards. Those who lived nearby would stop by on their lunch hours or after work to check on me. They saw me in my chicken cap and didn't mind when I asked, "Why don't you ever visit me?" even though they had stopped by the day before. I forgot things so easily with my chemo brain. These friends invited me to parties and luncheons even when they knew I might not be able to make it.

True friendship is unconditional, but the relationships were different because I was forced to show a weakness I had never shown before. I had to accept that I was human and not well. I was vulnerable. At the same time, I was able to show strength I had never shown before. I borrowed courage and strength from anyone who would give it, and that helped me maintain a sense of humor and a fighting spirit. In a strange way, my friendships helped me block out the possibility that cancer could kill me. Overall, I think my relationships with my true friends strengthened. Many friends told me that I was an inspiration to them. I hope that's true. Part of the credit goes to my friends for helping me to do that.

My relationship with strangers changed, too. When I met a stranger (not through my volunteer work where I am fully aware I will be talking about breast cancer) and the topic of breast cancer came up, I sometimes wished I could pull into a shell and hide. Sometimes I didn't want to talk about having breast cancer. I didn't want to be labeled.

At other times, I felt a need to foster relationships with strangers to let them know that breast cancer does affect young women. One day I went into a store and the store manager, who recognized me but was unaware of my cancer diagnosis, said, "So, is anything new with you?" I almost replied, "Well, as a matter of fact, the past few months have been really difficult. I had my last radiation treatment for breast cancer last week and I am really tired." But I didn't want to get into it. I just wanted to be a regular shopper. That's when it occurred to me that even my relationships with strangers had changed. Breast cancer is a fact that I can reveal or conceal, just like anything else that I can hide from others; but I cannot ignore it, even when I want to.

Even though I sometimes just want to be "ordinary," I believe that everything happens for a reason. I believe I have the potential to make a positive impact in the lives of people I meet. Simple acts of kindness are so important. Since being diagnosed with cancer, I have made a point of being kind to others—especially if I can remain anonymous during the process (such as paying for the car behind me on a toll road).

I know I can make a difference by sharing my experience of breast cancer with others. I almost always strike up conversations when I see someone wearing a pink ribbon breast cancer awareness pin. I ask about the pin and share my experience.

After I was diagnosed with breast cancer, I changed. Not just physically but also emotionally. And like other kinds of change, it has not always been easy. But it has been very rewarding. I cannot imagine what my life would be like if I were not a breast cancer survivor.

Jen

As a female, you spend a good part of your adolescence waiting for your breasts to make their grand entrance. Will they ever come in? Will they be too small? I've always been a size C cup, so I was satisfied. My breasts weren't too big. They weren't too small. I was feeling pretty good about my body. I wouldn't have minded slightly smaller hips or losing my double chin, but otherwise, I was in pretty decent shape. Then came breast cancer and the mastectomy, and I wasn't sure how I could ever feel sexy again.

I was pregnant when I had the mastectomy, so intimacy wasn't at the top of my list anyway. I was not one of those women who suddenly craved sex during pregnancy. I loved being pregnant and watching my body change, but after surgery, I had a very hard time adjusting to the loss of my breast. I even wore a camisole with light padding on the left side under my pajamas so that my chest would look symmetrical. I was trying to hide my new body from Matt. I wore my camisole during labor, too, because I did not want the medical staff to notice what I was missing.

After Parker was born, my body started returning to its normal shape. At my six-week check-up, the obstetrician gave us the green light to go ahead with our sex life, but I was not in a hurry. I was very nervous. I had been through a lot and wasn't sure how the experience would be. I wasn't comfortable with my missing breast, so I wore a tee shirt the entire time. Matt was so good to me. This wasn't something he had anticipated—his wife at age twenty-seven losing her breast—but he was fantastic. I mean, most men love breasts—although Matt always joked that he was more of a legs man; and I still had a decent set of legs. We both had to laugh the first time he went to touch two breasts, temporarily forgetting I had lost one. It took me several more times before I could be comfortable being intimate without wearing a shirt.

Another difficulty about intimacy was birth control. I wasn't able to take anything hormonally to prevent another pregnancy. Even though my tumor was estrogen-negative, my doctors did not want the estrogen levels in my body to increase. That meant no birth control pill, patch, or shot.

After getting pregnant with Parker so quickly, it was apparent that I was very fertile. Since my cycles had returned to a normal state, I assumed that I was still very fertile. I wasn't excited about the idea of an IUD (intrauterine device). Our only option was to start using condoms. After being married for five years, the last thing you think you will have to do is use a condom; nevertheless, Matt dutifully took on that responsibility. This is not a fantastic option, so we knew that once we had decided our family was complete, one of us would take care of this issue permanently.

It was hard for me to look at my old lingerie. I didn't wear it very much because I didn't fill it all out any more. Some of my coworkers had given me a gift certificate to Victoria's Secret as part of a care package. It was so sweet of them to think of me, but it was one of the last places I wanted to go with one breast. My new bras now had a special pocket for Boobsie so that she wouldn't pop out unexpectedly. I decided to go and see what else I might buy—underwear perhaps, or pajamas.

When I walked into the store and saw all the sexy bras and pictures of women with voluptuous breasts, I wanted to run. I quickly picked out some underwear and went to pay for it. A store promotion was offering customers something new each month, such as a bra or underwear. The saleswoman asked me whether I wanted some free lingerie. All I had to do was sign up. I politely told her I was not interested. Being a good salesperson, she tried to persuade me. I respectfully said no again. When she kept on, I finally blurted out, "I'm not interested because I had breast cancer and a mastectomy." She didn't know what to say. I paid and got the heck out of there. I'm sure she was embarrassed, but she couldn't have felt as bad as I did. It was a dose of reality. I might look normal with my clothes on, but when it came down to it, I was different from my friends, coworkers, and most women of my age, a fact that would become more apparent to me over time.

However, laughter truly is one of the best medicines. For example, Matt and I came up with some funny code names. After Boobsie got wet, she got a little heavy, so she tended to droop. We had a code for when I wanted to check whether I needed to make an adjustment at the pool. I'd say to Matt, "Even?" He'd reply, "Steven," if my breasts were symmetrical. If they needed some adjustment, he'd come up with a code word so I would know what to adjust. That way, other people had no idea what we were talking about.

Reconstruction has made a huge impact on my self-esteem. I feel more desirable. I hate it that it took getting a new set of boobs to feel that way, but it did. Reconstruction is a personal decision, but I am so happy I did it. It gave me back a piece of what was taken away five years before.

None of this is what we envisioned when we took our vows eleven years ago, but I cannot imagine going through this experience with anyone else. I am so fortunate that I had Matt by my side. I will never be able to repay him for his strength, his acceptance, and his love. An experience like this can either make or break a marriage. I used to think we needed nothing else to bring us closer, but somehow this has. I believe we can make it through anything now. Matt is my soulmate, and I am blessed beyond words.

My relationship with my parents was also enriched by this experience. As an only child, I was always very close to them. I suppose all three of us have had to acknowledge our mortality and cherish our moments together. When my mom was sixteen, her mother died from an allergic reaction to a penicillin shot. It was a complete shock to her entire family. When I was growing up, I dreaded turning sixteen because I was afraid my mom would die. Never did I think that it would be me who might not be around to raise my children.

It was only after becoming a parent myself that I understood the amazing love that my parents have for me. Seeing me sick and in pain must have been incredibly hard for them. As a child, you love your parents immensely. As a wife, you love your husband with an equal but different kind of love. But the love for your children is beyond comparison. As a parent, you will do anything for your child. Anything. It is unbearable to see your child hurt. As much as I know breast cancer hurt my parents, I am grateful for the strength they showed. No matter how old I am, I will always be their baby. I understand that now.

Parker gets upset with me when I recite from *Love You Forever* by Robert N. Munsch:

I'll love you forever,
I'll like you for always,
As long as I'm living
my baby you'll be.

He tells me that he is a big boy, not a baby. Some day he'll understand. I am thankful that I can appreciate my parents now while they are still living, and I look forward to the day when my children have their own children and can begin to understand how very much I love them.

I have to admit that I was nervous about my post–breast cancer relationships with my girlfriends. Some of my ZTA sisters and I decided to take a trip to the lake together a year and a half after my mastectomy. One of my girlfriends, Jill, was able to get her in-laws' lake house for the weekend. Seven of us were going, and though I looked forward to the time away, I was nervous about what to do. My swimsuit wouldn't be nearly as cute as everyone else's. No bikini for me. My swimsuit wasn't that bad, but I missed the days of being able to wear anything I wanted to.

I wasn't sure what to do at night, either. I had long gotten over the need to wear a camisole under my pajamas at home, but it was evident that a part of me was missing if I didn't wear it. At the lake house we were sharing bedrooms, and it wasn't very private. The first night, I wore my bra under my pajamas. Everyone else had their jammies on and bras off.

One of my girlfriends, Belinda, looked at me and quietly asked, "Do you have something on?" I explained that I had left my bra on so I wouldn't freak them out. Immediately, they all told me to do whatever I felt comfortable with, but they wished I would just be comfortable and take it off. So I decided to let these women, who had never seen me without Boobsie, in on my big secret. I took off my bra. This was a *big* step for me. I didn't want them to think of me differently, and they didn't.

The next day, out on the lake, we really bonded. We caught up on our lives—with happy marriages and failed marriages, careers, kids, and health issues. One of the more outgoing girls, Julie, told me she wanted to see my fake boob. The other girls did, too. So, there in a cove, I whipped out Boobsie and showed them. Their acceptance of me was just what I needed. I felt that even though I had changed in so many ways, I could still be "Jen" from college. Still outgoing and anally organized, but now more confident that they would still love me, no matter what my appearance was like.

I was also worried about work relationships and how breast cancer might affect my future career. I was very open with everyone at work. I wanted them to learn from my experience so that they would be aware that this does happen to healthy young women who have no family history of cancer. I didn't consider the possible consequences of being so open. I could have been seen as too much of a risk and been passed over for promotions. They could have been afraid that I would get sick again and not be able to perform my job.

But I am very fortunate; I found just the opposite. I was known as a hard worker before, and that has not changed. My coworkers seem to have even more respect for me because of all that I endured. I received a promotion a year after my diagnosis. I was relieved to be treated no differently. It was also scary. I didn't want to take on too much. I knew that I needed to stay as stress-free as possible for my health and for the sake of my family, so I have been strategic in my career moves. This is one of the best things about my breast cancer experience: I am able to take it all in stride because, in the end, there is nothing more important than my health, my family, and my relationship with God.

One of the most amazing benefits was my newfound relationships with other breast cancer survivors. I liken the bond to that of soldiers after a war. There are wounds so deep both physically and mentally that a "civilian" can't possibly understand the loss of a breast or a head of hair, that I have looked mortality in the face. The Nordie Girls have played a tremendous part in my healing. It is so comfortable being with them. I feel we are soulmates and that we have known each other far longer than a few years. I can tell them how I am feeling and they get it. They understand how I desperately want to be the same Jennifer Johnson I once was, yet I am forever changed. At our monthly luncheons, we joke that we are like the friends from *Sex and the City*, but we get to add breast cancer to our topics of conversation. And our sex lives aren't nearly as exciting as theirs.

In most of my relationships, things have basically remained the same. I think people have a new respect for me because of what I have been through; but at this point, I don't think they see me and think "breast cancer survivor." Breast cancer will always be a part of me, but it does not define me as a person. The greatest gift was learning to cherish all my relationships because none of us knows what tomorrow holds.

Kim

I never really gave much thought to breasts, particularly mine, until I was diagnosed with breast cancer. I was blessed with

ample-sized breasts—a C cup. I always had a nice figure and after my pregnancy I was able to still wear sexy, plunging neckline shirts or dresses on special occasions. I enjoyed feeling sexy
and feminine, and it never occurred to me that some day I
might not have my breasts. After I gave birth to Brandon, I was
focused mostly on losing the pudgy belly I had developed. Although having children changes your body forever in some
ways, mine was finally getting back to normal. All in all, I was
pleased with my body and my sexuality.

However, the minute I was diagnosed with breast cancer, it
hit me square in the face: We live in a breast-obsessed society.
Breasts are identified with sexuality in our society. For the first
time, I too was focused on breasts and on realizing that mine
would never be the same.

It is true—breasts are dispensable. You don't need them to
live. However, those biological facts seem insignificant when
you're talking about not having your own breasts anymore. I
chose to have reconstructive surgery so I would have a breast,
although it didn't look exactly like my other one. From the very
beginning, Scott was wonderful. Until then, I never knew how
strong our relationship and our marriage really was—physically,
emotionally, and spiritually. Scott helped change my bandages
and cared for me and my new breast from day one. But after seeing all that, I wondered whether he could ever find me sexy
again. I was angry because, before I was diagnosed, our sex life
was just getting back to normal after childbirth, and we were finally starting to have sex more than once every few months.
And then, bam! Breast cancer. I'm not saying that sex is the basis of our relationship, but for me, being sexual with the man I
love does play an important part.

During chemo, we didn't have much sex. I was too tired, and when I did have energy, I wanted to play with Brandon or just spend time with family and friends. Also, chemo affected my sex drive. I was so happy when I learned at a breast cancer conference that a potential side effect from treatment is loss of libido, even though that knowledge didn't change my situation. In addition, vaginal dryness and premature menopause, two other potential side effects of chemo, made sex uncomfortable for me for some time. (The best recommendation I got from a fellow survivor was Astro Glide.)

The good news is that these side effects were only temporary. But that didn't stop me from worrying about Scott. I was his wife and I should be meeting his needs, but I couldn't do it. This fact caused a great deal of anxiety and made me feel like a failure as a wife at times. Scott would joke with me and say that he could take care of his needs in the shower. While I was undergoing chemo, Scott did hold me a lot, and that was as good as sex at that point in my life. Scott knew I wanted affection and love, but I was not ready for sex, and he knew exactly what to say and how to meet my needs.

After my reconstruction, I was afraid to have sex. The first time was like the first time after giving birth to Brandon. I was scared and tense. I was also afraid that Scott would not want to touch me. I had always enjoyed foreplay, but now I wasn't sure whether Scott would want to touch me or whether I would be able to feel him touching me on my breasts or stomach.

After my reconstruction, I was able to wear my sexy shirts, and even lingerie. Unfortunately, my old underwire bras irritated my scars so I had to find bras with no underwire. It's not easy to find sexy bars with no underwire. My old swimsuits fit me fine, but I couldn't wear them because of the scar across my stomach, which went from hip to hip (my smiley face). The scar across my abdomen had more of an effect on me than my new boob. I know it's my battle scar, and with time I know it will fade, but it's a constant reminder to me. I had to purchase new swimsuits and new jeans. No more low-riders. And I don't feel very sexy in my underwear because of the scar. I refuse to wear "grandma" underwear at this point.

After my treatments ended, my sexual desire didn't come back for a while. And, like Jen, I was frustrated with the birth control situation. We were advised not to try to have children for at least three to five years. My doctor wouldn't let me take birth control pills, so we had to use condoms. Frankly, using condoms was an inconvenience. We were married—we shouldn't have to use them. Sometimes, using a condom ruined the moment for me and would bring me back to the reality that I had cancer and shouldn't get pregnant right now. Once, the condom broke while we were having sex. I was freaked out and started crying. I kept saying, "I can't be pregnant. I don't want the cancer to come back." Needless to say, this experience ruined the moment.

Now four years after my diagnosis, I am happy to report that my sex drive is back. I still feel the need to be intimate. I want affection. I need to be touched. And I actually enjoy sex again; no longer do I think about cancer or my boobs. I feel free again.

Scott is my true hero in all of this. He and I have an amazing partnership and have leaned on each other so much in times of crisis. We've been together since we were fifteen years old and we have always been there for each other. He always knows just what to do or say. I think our relationship has been strengthened by the breast cancer experience. We talk even more openly about things and share what's on our minds. I never knew I could love him more than I already did, but after this experience, words can't describe how deeply I love him. I feel that our love has been renewed and is so much more powerful now. Together, I feel we can accomplish anything.

Like the other Nordie Girls, my breast cancer experience also changed my relationships with my friends and my family in a positive way. I am convinced that I would not have been able to make it through my treatments without my family and friends. Having their unconditional love and support was critical for me. They were there for me every step of the way—the prayers (I have never believed more strongly in the power of prayer than now), the hats (my great friends held a hat party right before I lost my hair), the wonderful food (meals brought to our home for eight months), the house cleaning, the flowers, the cards, the e-mails, the phone calls, the visits . . . all were so supportive.

My relationship with my parents, who continue to inspire me by the way they live their own lives, was also strengthened through my experience with breast cancer. I have always been very close to them, and we've had an honest, open relationship. It was particularly difficult for my dad because I was his little girl, the same little girl he continues to call every Thursday and Sunday. My mom always knew just what to say and what to do. I think both my mom and my dad were proud of how I fought and how I became an advocate for breast cancer awareness. My brothers and their families were amazing as well. After my diagnosis, my ten-year-old niece even cut her long hair for the Locks of Love charity, which provides wigs to children going through cancer. I think my cancer diagnosis made my entire family face the reality of mortality and appreciate the time that we do have together. This was particularly poignant when my Aunt Barbara passed away from breast cancer two years after I was diagnosed.

My two best friends, Laura and Kristin, always knew what to say and do. Kristin, a nurse by training, would help with my bandages. She was also my chemo angel, showering me with gifts and a nice lunch after every treatment. And Laura would drive four hours with her two boys in the car just to make sure she was at my surgeries. These two friends, who are truly my sisters, made me realize how lucky I was. And there were dozens of other friends just like them.

My breast cancer helped me realize that time is precious. I now try to eliminate things in my life that drain my energy. Sometimes, that has meant a friendship or a relationship. Life is too short to surround myself with negative people. Breast cancer has given me the courage to realize this.

I have chosen to build a soulful community. Part of that community has come from knowing other breast cancer survivors. We've all been in the trenches, have faced our mortality, and are surviving and thriving in our own ways. These inspiring men and women gave me hope when I needed it most.

And then, there are the Nordie Girls. These women—Patti, Jana, and Jen—opened up their hearts to me from the instant I met them. They answered my questions, gave me advice and support—and most of all—gave me unconditional love. These women understood what I was going through and were willing to share their lessons and their stories. The

Nordie Girls continue to be a source of strength for me, and their friendship is something that I truly cherish.

So, my relationships changed after breast cancer—they became deeper. Today, I'm not afraid to say what I'm feeling. I hold on tight to my family and friends, and I cherish every minute because tomorrow is never promised. I truly feel I am a better person because of my breast cancer experience.

CHAPTER NINE

Motherhood

—— *Nordie's Café* ——
February 2003

Today the café was already crowded when Patti arrived to claim the coveted corner booth. In the center of the café, several tables were pushed together. Strollers and shopping bags were everywhere, as were booster seats and highchairs. The noise level was high—a dissonance of toddlers, crying babies, and women laughing.

When Jen arrived, she made her way around the tangle of children. Her belly was beginning to show, and she was radiant with her new "pregnancy glow." She excitedly exclaimed, "Only two more months to go!"

"My five-year plan includes being a mom," said Patti. "Even if that means adopting a child before I get married."

"It sure is loud in here today," commented Jana, as she arrived with Kim. The others chuckled. They were aware of her ambivalence about kids. Despite having worked part-time at a daycare center when she was in college (and she loved every minute of it), Jana was undecided about motherhood.

Kim had no such qualms. "It's a challenge to raise a child, but it's also rewarding. I love being a mom."

And so, against the backdrop of sporadic tantrums from children in the "Mommy and Me" party, the Nordie Girls confided how their treatments for breast cancer had impacted their future as mothers—or not.

Patti

I was told that about four months into my second chemo cycle my ovaries would dry up and shrivel to uselessness (this was not stated in those exact terms, but when you're twenty-seven and have no kids, that was essentially the message). However, several months into chemotherapy for my recurrence, a CT scan showed that my ovaries were firing stronger than before. In fact, a special note on the scan results stated that although most of my organs had stayed the same, the size of the small cysts in my ovaries had decreased. This fact, coupled with my healthier eating, must have explained my five-day cycle, which came complete with cramps.

Two months later, I was having periods again. However, the monthly visits from "Aunt Flo" would last for only a couple of hours rather than the usual week. This cycle surprised my oncologist. She was sure that my ovaries would "take a nap" after we started my new chemo regimen, and she nodded when I confirmed that "Flo" had not visited the previous month. (Score one: oncologist. Score one: ovaries. For those of you keeping score!)

My oncologist wanted me to take medicine that would completely shut down my ovaries. That night, I tossed and turned, realizing that I had not at all processed what it meant to go through menopause before my mother did. The night before my appointment, I lay in bed and cried as I thought about my friends who'd gotten pregnant and now had beautiful children. Would I ever experience the joy of pregnancy and having children?

I began making a list of pros and cons.

Pros of no childbirth:

- My tummy tuck would last forever.
- My hips wouldn't widen.
- I could still be a mother through adoption.
- The biggie: Sealing off my hormones would give the big "C" its final gut punch.

Cons:

- The obvious one: There would be no pregnancy and no child that was part me.
- I would never feel a baby kicking in my womb.
- I would have no excuse to shop for new clothes.

Okay, the last one isn't too important. Conceptually, my ovaries would only be asleep and could be awakened. But realistically, after my eggs and ovaries had toxic chemicals pumped into them for more than a year, what were the odds of their being healthy, thriving eggs? So I figured the likelihood of becoming pregnant and carrying a child full-term was slim. And besides, I was plain tired of cancer. Anything I could do to rid myself of it appealed to me.

So I kept my appointment and took the shot to put my ovaries to sleep; I pledged that I would not let my life change in any way other than throwing away my supply of tampons and pads. After the shot (actually it was a pellet in my abdomen), I walked out into the sunshine and decided to go on with my life. I was sure that there would be additional mourning when I got married and maybe wanted children with my future spouse, but I decided to work through that grief when the time came.

The additional mourning came sooner than expected. A few days later, I stopped at the bagel shop on my way to work for my morning treat (a bagel with light cream cheese). Inside, I saw a mother and daughter buying a dozen bagels. The little blonde girl was so cute, and she had the same eyes and cheeks as her mother. Suddenly, it hit me: No one in my future would have my eyes or hair. No one! The tears started before I reached the car with my bagel. By the time I got to the turn-off for work, I was a wreck.

Previously, in times like this, I would go shopping and spend a huge amount of money to make myself feel better—there's nothing like retail therapy. But now that thought got me even more upset because I realized that in the past I had used shopping to heal whatever was going on in my life that was unpleasant. Worse yet, I was a shopping addict who, instead of working through her issues, used purchasing power to deal with them. Finally, I had given up my credit card for Lent.

Later, I realized that this emotional roller coaster must have been the sign of menopause—but at the time I thought, "So now I'm a completely irrational woman, with no kids, no credit cards . . . and mascara running down what once was my perfectly balanced face."

What did I do to feel better? I took the Guy Forsythe CD out of my CD player and put in Jay Z; nothing like a little

filthy-word rap to help you feel better. Then I stopped at Mc-
Donald's for a Diet Coke. Usually, I give up soda for Lent; now
I was glad I had given up credit cards instead. The smiling man
at the window made me laugh, and I drove out of McDonald's
sipping soda and singing along to "Hustler," bad words and all.

Experiences such as this made me feel as if I were going
through PMS and menopause at the same time. I suppose I
was simply adjusting to my hormone treatment. You don't realize that hormones are such an integral part of you until
they're taken away. Most women lose their hormones gradually. Mine were gone in an instant.

It is "very rare," according to my doctor, for someone to
continue to have her menstrual cycle after undergoing months
of chemotherapy and then to have PMS and menopause at
the same time. In the words of my oncologist, who calmed me
after I called her and hysterically told her that I was attempt-
ing the impossible (simultaneous PMS and menopause):
"Chill out, and we'll worry about it if it happens again next
month . . . "

As for motherhood, watching a friend adopt a beautiful
child made the prospect of adoption more real to me. My sce-
nario had me adopting two cute little Chinese girls. As for losing hormones . . . well, I wouldn't wish it on anyone. But I
adjusted, realizing that it was all part of my big fight with the
big "C."

Jana

As soon as I got married, the questions began: "So, when are
you and Chris going to have children?" This age-old question
is not unique to us. All newlyweds seem to be fair game. And

everyone has a different level of acceptance of the question. Some share their excitement about family planning. Others avoid answering it at all. As for me, I am personally sensitive to the question. With the reality of cancer focusing my attention on saving my own life, thoughts of creating a new life left me ambivalent about motherhood.

After my initial diagnosis, I asked one of my oncologists whether I'd be able to have children after chemotherapy, and if so, when? I was told that if my health "looked good" after five years, the oncologist would "endorse" my having children. This rationale was based on this oncologist's thought that a cancer patient is "not out of the woods" until after five years, and that to have a child and risk dying at a young age would not be fair to the child. Physically, I could safely become pregnant as early as one to two years after chemotherapy ended if the chemotherapy had not affected my menstrual cycles and fertility.

During those two years, I was concerned about unintentional pregnancy. Especially since I could no longer take birth control pills because they contained the female hormones that fed my ER/PR positive tumor. Later, when the Zoladex I was on caused premature menopause, my fear abated.

When Chris and I were dating, we had "the talk" about whether we wanted children or not, and if so, how many, and when. Neither of us felt strongly about becoming parents, and this added assurance about our compatibility.

When my breast cancer metastasized, Chris and I had a decision to make—should we pull out all the stops to try to save my life, knowing that some of the treatments would rule out having natural children of our own, or should we risk my health by trying to have a child and hope for the best? Chris

was adamant that we focus on saving my life. And, having discussed parenthood previously, we knew that adoption was an
option if we ever wanted to become parents. Right now, Chris
continues to tell me that our "couplehood life" is abundant
and fulfilling, and I agree.

The treatment regimen recommended for my metastatic
breast cancer would shut down my ovaries either chemically
or with a hysterectomy. I opted for the chemical treatment.

The drug used, Zoladex, pushed me into full-blown premature menopause. The "good" thing is that I no longer worry
about menstrual cramps, bloating, fatigue, or birth control.
The "bad" things are the hot flashes, moodiness, and weight
gain, and possibly an increased risk for other health issues later
in life, such as heart disease and osteoporosis.

With every hot flash I got, Chris exclaimed, "It's working!"
It was his way of turning a negative event into a positive one.
But apparently the hot flashes were not working, because three
years after starting premature menopause, the cancer metastasized into my chest wall. Now I just wish the hot flashes would
burn calories (after all, they're often described by other women
as "power surges," and they really make me feel as if I were having a workout). I'm frustrated by the forty pounds I have gained
since my premature menopause started.

Also, each hot flash reminds me that natural parenthood is
not an option. I tell myself that I'm relieved about not having
to worry about getting pregnant, because I don't have strong
urges to become a mother; but a small part of me does wonder what would it be like to have new life growing inside me
that is half me and half Chris. It's an experience I will never
have.

Jen

My first early lesson as a mother and a breast cancer survivor
hit me in the face. I couldn't breast-feed Parker, at least not immediately because I had just completed chemotherapy. I could
begin three weeks after my last treatment. Until then, I had to
pump and throw away the milk I produced.

After all that I'd been through, I wasn't sure about breast-
feeding anyway; but I thought I should give it a try, so I purchased a pump and began trying to produce milk. After four
days, I threw in the towel. This cow (that's what I felt like) was
just not producing. I guess my body had been through too
much trauma. I have since found that other young survivors in
similar situations have also faced a lack of milk.

But if I wasn't able to nurse, how would I make it in other
mothering situations? Would I ever figure out how to sew a
costume? Or help Parker create a masterpiece for his science
project? After this line of self-questioning, finally, I began to
laugh. I was putting way too much pressure on myself.

I believe it was another sign from God that I needed to take
it easy and let Matt and my family help me with Parker. It was
more exhausting to get up every few hours to feed a baby than
I had anticipated. Matt was wonderful, and we took turns at
night. A relative of ours who worked for a baby formula manu-
facturer sent us a huge shipment of formula, which was very
helpful financially. Formula is expensive!

Two life-changing experiences had happened to me at the
same time. I brought a child into this world and faced my own
mortality. Either one would have been a challenge on its own;
facing both at the same time was pretty overwhelming.

In many ways, it was good. I learned to slow down and appreciate the little moments with Parker. In other ways, I felt a bit cheated out of his youth and mine. I spent too much of Parker's first year worrying. Will I be around to raise him? I felt as if I had to cram a lifetime of love into a very short time, and it angered me. Why couldn't I have an idyllic experience with my child?

Now that more than five years have passed, I am thankful. My end-of-treatment anniversary is the day before Parker's birthday, so each year his birthday is a double blessing: He is a year older, and I am one more year away from this disease.

Being a mother is the most rewarding—and challenging—thing I have ever done. I have a "boss" to whom I am on call twenty-four hours a day. I am his live-in chef, nurse, comforter, teacher, and provider. Best of all, I am the recipient of his love. I never imagined how my life would be so completely turned upside down by having a child. I certainly did not anticipate this type of love.

I could go on and on about the thrills of all Parker's firsts— the first time he ate solid food, the first time he crawled, the first time he walked—I was filled with happiness to enjoy each of these moments, as any normal mom would be.

The further out I got from my diagnosis, the more I allowed myself to think about being around the next few years. I became more confident in my body again, and Matt and I began talking about having a second child.

Did we have enough love for a second child? Would we be cheating Parker? Would a new child be healthy? And how would another pregnancy affect my health? A minority of breast cancer patients are younger than forty, so there isn't a lot of data on pregnancy after breast cancer. When doctors cautioned me to wait from two to five years before trying again, that was fine with Matt and me. I wasn't sure I could mentally handle a potential recurrence during another pregnancy.

Matt and I had always planned to have at least two children, maybe three. The doctors told me that surgery would not hamper my fertility, but chemotherapy might. I was so focused on trying to live for the child in my womb that I would have done anything—even if it meant losing my fertility in the future.

At my two-year (posttreatment) appointment, I brought up the question of having a second child. My oncologist raised his brow a bit and said, "The longer you wait, the happier I'll be." It is believed that women with estrogen-receptor positive cancers may be at a higher risk for dormant cancer cells to become active again because of hormone surges during pregnancy. My tumor was estrogen-receptor negative, but it was slightly positive for progesterone, which is also elevated during pregnancy. I also wondered what effects chemo would have on remaining eggs. What about possible birth defects? There just wasn't enough data to help me make a decision. My oncologist did share with me a study showing that pregnancy after breast cancer can have a "healthy mother effect." Many questions were still unanswered, but I was encouraged because pregnancy after breast cancer did not seem to increase the likelihood of a recurrence.

My surgeon, on the other hand, said she thought it would be fine to think about adding to our family now that I was two years out. I was a little surprised, but excited at the thought.

Serious "baby pains" hit about six months later when we were in Arkansas visiting my family and I watched Parker playing with his cousins. I told Matt about my feelings, but after talking about it for several weeks, we decided to wait another year before trying. We'd be at a better place financially, and I'd be four years out from my diagnosis.

Shortly after this grand decision, I realized my cycle was late. My cycles were otherwise like clockwork. After five more days, I picked up a pregnancy test. Sure enough, the test turned blue. I was pregnant! Matt and I had used a condom faithfully—except once. That's all it took. Obviously, chemotherapy had not affected my fertility.

The first person I contacted was my surgeon, who was so happy for me. I felt instantly more at ease. Her confidence that this was wonderful news was just what I needed. She said that she would follow me closely during the pregnancy with visits every two months to monitor things. This made me feel that if something did show up, we would catch it early.

I shared my news with the Nordie Girls at our next lunch. I knew they would understand how excited and scared I was, both at the same time. They were thrilled. "We're having a baby!" exclaimed Patti.

We told Matt's mom first. She didn't seem worried about the health issue. A few weeks later at a dinner to celebrate my thirtieth birthday, we told my parents. I was so nervous about breaking the news that I waited until after we had left the restaurant and reached home again—just in case they freaked out. But they took the news very well. Mom said she'd been wondering if we were thinking about another baby.

The pregnancy was going smoothly, but I was into my sixteenth week of pregnancy when I felt a lump in my right breast. This couldn't happen again?

I panicked and called my surgeon's office. She didn't think it felt like a cancerous tumor, but she went ahead and performed an ultrasound. Everything looked good. She told me to stop touching it and to come back in four weeks.

It was so hard not to touch the lump. I obsessed over it. But four weeks later, the lump had disappeared. And the rest of my pregnancy went smoothly.

One night, Parker asked me where my belly was. I told him and said, "That's where the baby is." "Is that your belly, too?" He pointed to my chest.

"No. That's mommy's chest. Her boobies."

A little later we went upstairs to bed. I was changing into pajamas when Parker walked in. He said, "Mommy, where's your boobie?" He could see that I was missing my breast, so I explained that I had an "owie," but the doctors had made it all better. So now I had one real booby and one pretend booby.

A few weeks later, we were at a restaurant for Sunday brunch. In a loud voice, Parker proclaimed, "Mommy has one 'fortend' boobie and one real boobie." ("Fortend" was his word for "pretend.") We couldn't help but laugh, but it made me wonder what he was telling the kids at his preschool.

After an uneventful pregnancy, I was three weeks from my due date when I felt a sensation of warm fluid. Had my water broken? No way! I had just seen the doctor that day and had not felt any labor pains. The doctor on-call told me to go to the hospital and check it out. I couldn't reach Matt or my mom, so a friend drove me. My water had broken. Once again, I was having a baby with no warning!

Five hours after my water broke, Matt and I welcomed Emma Grace into our lives. She had a full head of dark hair and beautiful blue eyes. And I'd survived natural childbirth.

I decided I wanted to try nursing, even if I could do it only from one side. If women can breast-feed twins, I thought, I can breast-feed a baby from one breast. It was comical at the hospital. Though I'd made it clear that I had only one breast, the lactation consultant at first tried hard to find a breast on both sides.

I just put old Boobsie into a nursing bra and it worked great. I breast-fed Emma for six months from one breast, supplementing with formula. I am so thankful for the opportunity to breast-feed. Although painful in the beginning, it was a wonderful bonding experience and it allowed me to see my breast as something beautiful again.

Now that we have Emma, our family feels complete. I worry sometimes about both of my kids' risk for breast cancer, especially Emma's. When she was three months old, I noticed a knot under her right nipple. "It's nothing," I told myself, but I called the pediatrician right away. The nurses assured me it was perfectly normal. My hormones could stay in her system for a while. I showed it to Emma's pediatrician at her four-month visit. She knew about the breast cancer and understood my concern, but she, too, assured me that it was nothing.

I tried not to look for it every time I dressed Emma, but I was always aware of it and always a little freaked out. It disappeared when she was around ten months old. I was so relieved.

I asked my surgeon when we should start checking Emma for breast cancer. I'd heard it should be ten years earlier than your mother's age at diagnosis, which would mean seventeen for her, but my surgeon said we would probably start around age twenty. So I try not to focus too much on cancer "what-ifs" because I don't want to miss the innocence of Emma's childhood. In twenty years, I tell myself, the medical community may have found a cure, and it will certainly have made great progress.

After my breast cancer experience, I started collecting items for my kids for the big moments in their lives and kept them in a special drawer. Matt knows where the drawer is, and I label things just in case I don't get to give the gifts to them myself. If I find a card or something special I want them to have on their graduation or wedding days, I buy it now. It makes me feel better to have it on hand—partly because I am a planner and partly because they will know that I care about them and am with them on those special days no matter what happens to me or what the future holds.

One of the most rewarding milestones I reached was Parker's first day of kindergarten last year. Tears for moms and even dads are a normal part of the first day, but none of the other parents could have imagined how amazing it was that either of us, much less both of us, had lived to reach this milestone. As I walked away from Parker's classroom, I couldn't help but thank God over and over for letting me live to experience this day.

Recently I attended a conference sponsored by Living Beyond Breast Cancer and the Young Survival Coalition. After hearing about other women survivors who desperately wanted children but weren't sure whether they could or should have them, I understood how fortunate I am.

I never take my two miracles for granted. I hope that my being able to have a child after breast cancer gives hope to other young women.

Kim

The moment I heard "You have breast cancer," I thought about Scott and how he would raise Brandon all alone without me in the picture. It scared me to death. Scott is an amazing father and he would do an exceptional job, but this was not what we had signed up for. We are a team. We are lifelong partners. We are parents who want to be together watching Brandon put a corsage on his prom date, graduating from high school and college, and marrying the love of his life. We are supposed to become grandparents together so that we can spoil our grandchildren rotten and then send them home to their parents.

During my treatments, Brandon kept me going. No matter how sick I felt from chemotherapy or how much pain I was in from my surgery, if I looked into Brandon's smiling face, my pain and fear would go away. On those days when I felt too tired to climb the stairs, or even to eat, I saw Brandon's smile. On days when I really didn't want to go for my treatment, I saw Brandon's smile. And on those days when I just didn't think I would make it, I saw Brandon's smile.

Motherhood is amazing. I never knew I could love another human being so much. The whole concept of giving birth and bringing another person into this world is a gift from God, and Brandon was exactly that—a beautiful gift from God.

Thinking that Brandon might grow up without me made me angry with God at first. Then I decided that instead of being angry, I needed to be happy for the time I had with Brandon right now. Before my cancer diagnosis, I was a spiritual person, but not one who prayed every night. Now, I pray. I thank God for today and ask for one more day.

I pray, "God, please let me see my son grow up. He needs me. Scott needs me. Don't take me away now. I will be here to serve you. Just give me one more day."

Scott and I always wanted children, although we disagreed about how many. I wanted two: a boy and a girl. Scott wanted three. Scott and I have been together since we were freshmen in high school. We had been married for six years when we decided it was time to start our family. We took a weekend vacation trip, had unprotected sex once, and voila—I was pregnant. Just call me Fertile Myrtle. Brandon arrived a month early and was in the neonatal intensive care unit for a week. I held him for the first time on Valentine's Day, two days after he was born. Exactly two years later on Valentine's Day, I started my first round of chemotherapy treatment, this time fighting for my own life.

Being a mother who is undergoing treatment for breast cancer is no easy task. Not only are there emotional issues about whether you're going to live to raise your son but also there are the physical realities. There were times when I was so tired that I felt I couldn't take care of Brandon the way a mom should. I also felt robbed of special moments with him, although this made me appreciate more the moments we did have together.

"Just in case," I wanted to make a video that Brandon could watch at important points in his life—turning sixteen, graduation day, wedding day, first job, birth of his children. I got the idea from the movie My Life, which I had watched ten years earlier in college. The movie was about a dying father who shot a video for his unborn son. At the end of the movie, my friends were bawling their eyes out, but I felt a weird sense of peace. When they asked why I wasn't crying, I said it was because the dad had left his son a beautiful gift. Was that a premonition of what was to come for me ten years later?

Unfortunately, Scott didn't see it the same way and refused to make the video. "You are not going to die anytime soon," he said. Although I agree with him now, I still want to make my video for Brandon. In the meantime, I have written letters to him. And I make a point of being in more of our family video footage.

After cancer, I had a hard time focusing on my career. I never thought I was a stay-at-home mom, but now I realize how quickly time goes by, and I don't want to miss any of my son's life. A line from the movie *Steel Magnolias* comes to mind. Julia Roberts's character, Shelby, was risking her life to get pregnant, and she said to her mother: "I would rather have thirty minutes of wonderful than a lifetime of nothing special." That's exactly how I feel.

Right now I feel so blessed to have one healthy child that I worry we might be pressing our luck to want another one. My breast cancer history, along with the possibility that Scott and I could be carriers of a rare genetic disorder, seems to be asking for trouble. Also, I had a rough pregnancy with Brandon. Can my body handle another pregnancy?

As Jen pointed out, there are simply not enough studies about the effects of chemotherapy on fertility. When I learned I had breast cancer and asked about the fertility issue, none of my doctors had answers. What they did tell me was that the chemotherapy could cause me to go into early-onset menopause and the chances of having my own children could be destroyed.

Some young women who are diagnosed with cancer have their eggs harvested before they start chemo. I had already begun chemo when I learned about egg harvesting, so this wasn't an option for me. In hindsight, I wish I would have researched these options before I started chemotherapy. Fortunately, there is a great organization called Fertile Hope that educates cancer patients about these options.

When I went in for my two-year check-up, my doctor gave me the green light: I could start trying to get pregnant again.

Fortunately for me, I was estrogen/progesterone-receptor negative, so there were fewer concerns about hormone surges during pregnancy. Although my periods had stopped during chemotherapy, my menstrual cycle had come back, and I was now experiencing regular monthly periods. This was good news.

The thought of trying to get pregnant and have another child made me feel excited and scared. What if my cancer comes back? I know that Scott could handle raising Brandon alone, but what about two children? Would that be fair to him? Then I realized that I can't live in fear. I have to trust that God will lead us in the right direction. Jen and many other women have gone on to bear healthy babies after breast cancer. That fact gave me the hope and courage I needed.

When I look at Brandon, I realize that motherhood is such an amazing thing; for this reason, Scott and I have decided that we want to have another child. If we can't have our own children naturally, we will look into adoption. And regardless of what happens, I feel blessed that I have experienced motherhood. God definitely played a hand in giving us Brandon when he did.

Four years after my diagnosis, I also was able to see a milestone in Brandon's life—his first day of kindergarten. When I was first diagnosed with breast cancer, I was not sure I would be there for that special day—but I was. It was a bittersweet day for me. Many of the mothers were in tears—their babies were heading to school—all grown up. I was in tears—but for a different reason. I was blessed to be here to see Brandon on this special day. Yes, I was sad that he was growing up so fast, but I was alive and there, and that's what mattered.

Now that I'm officially four years out from my cancer diagnosis, I have decided to undergo genetic testing. Genetic testing is available for two of the identified breast cancer genes, BRCA 1 and BRCA 2. I wanted to do the testing before we started trying to have another child. If a woman carries the BRCA 1 or BRCA 2 gene, she has an increased risk of breast and ovarian cancer during her lifetime. This may affect our decision about whether to have more children as well as about preventive measures.

The genetic testing, a simple blood test, showed that I am not a BRCA 1 or BRCA 2 gene carrier. Now I feel comfortable going ahead and trying to have another child. We are ready to start trying to expand our family. We'll see what God has in store for us.

Two Weeks

— *Nordie's Café* —
March 2003

Patti's seat was vacant. It was not the last Tuesday of the month—our normal meeting day. Instead we were meeting on a Monday—in the middle of the month. The clink of glasses and spoons that normally complemented the tinkle of our banter went unnoticed. Unlike past months, we wondered how to start the conversation.

The unspoken reality shared by all was that from this point forward, Patti's seat would be empty. The sadness of this reality had begun to sink in. We tried to make sense of it. Thoughts about the past week's events spun in our heads.

Shortly after our last luncheon, Patti's health had worsened. Her chemotherapy stopped working. Her liver started to shut down, and she went into the hospital. We knew that Patti's oncologist had met with her and her family and told them that she was out of treatment options.

We began talking and soon decided that if Patti could not come to Nordie's, we would take Nordie's to her in the form of her favorite dessert, chocolate mousse cake. This made us feel only slightly better. We tried to think of a gift we could take to her. Jana recalled a picture taken of the four of us at the Ribbons

& Racquets (R&R) fund-raising event several months earlier. Kim and Jen agreed that this was a perfect gift.

We purchased a metal frame and had "Nordie's at Noon" engraved on the top and our names "Jana Patti Kim Jen" on the bottom.

After hugging each other tightly, we said our good-byes. Each of us knew that our dream of sitting around "our" table at Nordie's as gray-haired, forty-year breast cancer survivors would not happen. How could we come to terms with the reality that our dear friend was dying?

Jana

Saturday

"I have a lot to do in two weeks!" proclaimed Patti when she called me shortly after six o'clock on a Saturday evening in March. She was calling from her hospital bed. Unbeknownst to the Nordie Girls, she'd been admitted a few days earlier. In the next day or so, she would go home to her apartment under Hospice care.

She told me all this in her usual casual, matter-of-fact manner. Her tone made Hospice sound as simple as bringing home a new television or a piece of furniture, and that I should stop by and check it out. Hospice! It was Patti's tactful, indirect way of telling me she was going home to die—in the next two weeks.

Patti's liver failure had reached the point where she was unable to eat. She could ingest only fluids. However, the fluids did not hydrate her, because they were not absorbed into her bloodstream; instead, they accumulated in her abdomen, making her dehydrated. As her liver failure worsened, it put stress on her kidneys. Once the liver (or any organ) shuts down, a domino effect begins: All the other organs shut down, the result being death.

I wished Patti goodnight, told her that I loved her and would see her soon. Then I hung up the phone and burst into tears. As I sobbed, I told Chris the news. He put his arms around me, which calmed me enough to call Jen. Jen offered to call Kim.

Sunday

On Sunday, I spoke to Patti's good friend Donna, who told me that Patti would probably go home on Tuesday, and that we (Jen, Kim, and I) could visit her there. Donna also told me that it might be possible for us to visit Patti in the hospital, but currently her family was being very selective about visitors. Patti needed to rest in anticipation of going home.

I passed on the news to Jen, who called Kim, and we waited for Tuesday. We also decided to meet for lunch at Nordie's the next day so that the three of us could support one another.

Later that day, Chris and I went to the florist where we found some miniature purple tulips and a long, narrow basket that looked almost like a window box. We arranged the flowers ourselves, and were pleased when the end result looked like "spring," Patti's favorite season. Then we dropped off our flowers and a card at the hospital's front desk.

Even though Patti received several flower arrangements and cards, she told me later that she especially appreciated having "spring" in her hospital room. I hold small memories like this close to my heart. It helps me handle the bittersweetness of those difficult two weeks.

Monday

When I spoke to Donna on Monday morning, she told me again that the Nordie Girls should plan on visiting Patti Tuesday evening. I called Jen, who called Kim. Then I drove to work. But I was very distracted. I couldn't focus. My mind kept drifting to Patti and what she had to do in the next "two weeks." Part of me couldn't believe that this was happening. I prayed for a miracle. "Let her recover and be just fine." Although I do believe miracles can occur, I knew from my nurse's training that I was in the denial stage of grief over Patti's dying.

Jen and Kim asked whether Patti's going home with Hospice care meant what they thought it meant. I explained that Hospice professionals and trained volunteers help patients and their families and friends prepare a comfortable setting in which the patient can live out his or her remaining days on earth. I didn't know much about the details, but had always heard that Hospice services were invaluable to families. I also knew that Hospice was never approved by insurance companies until someone truly was near the end of life or gravely ill.

About an hour after our lunch, Donna called me at work. Her voice was shaky as she told me we should come to the hospital at once to see Patti. The family had approved our visit and would be expecting us. Hurriedly, I called Jen, who called Kim, and we agreed to meet at the hospital within the next hour. "Not good news," I thought.

I ran home to get the picture of the four of us and meanwhile Kim picked up the engraved frame from the shop. Thank goodness it was ready. We wanted to give it to Patti now be-cause we all feared this would be our last chance to see her.

As we searched for Patti's room on the hospital's fifth floor, I remembered that I had recovered from my mastectomy on this very floor. My throat tightened at the memory. Then we saw Patti's parents and her brother, who had flown in from the East Coast; they were inside Patti's room, talking to a chaplain.

When we saw her, Patti tried to smile and be cheerful, but her eyes were lackluster and sunken; they had lost their trade-mark gleam. She was very frail and extremely pale. I was blind-sided by the reality. Patti's going to die! My throat tightened again. I tried to act normally, but what was normal in such a situation?

Underneath Patti's smile as she greeted us, I sensed a despon-dence, which I attributed to her acceptance that her end was near. She had fought the good battle, and for quite some time she had beaten the odds. Now she was preparing for her life af-ter death. This was my perception, but as we began to talk, it was apparent that Patti wasn't throwing in the towel just yet. She still had her fighting spirit, and there were some things she wanted to do in the next two weeks.

I wondered, though, whether she would even make it through the night. And although Patti had released everything to God, I was not ready to release her. I prayed she would have the extra days she wanted to accomplish whatever she needed to do.

Tuesday

Patti did go home as planned, and Hospice had arranged for a hospital bed and other medical equipment to be waiting at her "city apartment," as she affectionately called her home. Her

brother David had set up her living room with the hospital
bed in the middle surrounded by chairs and a futon.

Jen, Kim, and I were on the "guest list" for Tuesday evening,
part of round two of the scheduled visitors. Round one was
just ending, and it included several of her close friends from
work and college. David had arranged for a maximum number
of visitors at a time so that Patti would not be overwhelmed,
an arrangement that allowed each visitor ample time with her.
He was very good at hosting everyone while protecting his
older sister. Coordinating schedules gave him something productive to do, something to assuage his grief. Besides, someone
needed to coordinate Patti's many visitors.

That evening, our primary goal was to tape record Patti's responses to remaining questions about topics for our book.
Completing *Nordie's at Noon* was high on her list of priorities,
and she had made it clear that we were to pursue publication.
She also gave approval for us to interview her friends and family, and she agreed that David could assist with writing her remaining chapters, if necessary.

During our final interview, I felt a sense of peace in the
midst of what would otherwise be an extraordinarily awkward
setting. Several candles were lit. Patti's Christmas decorations
were still up (even though it was March), including Christmas cards on the walls. When I commented on the cards,
Patti said Christmas was her favorite holiday; she kept the
cards displayed because they reminded her of how many
people loved her.

That evening, Patti looked much better than the day before
in the hospital. She had more energy and her skin color was
better; however, that may have been due to a difference in

lighting. Also, the twinkle was back in her eyes. I thought she just might make it two more weeks!

Wednesday

My older sister, Angi, was Patti's hair stylist at this time, so Angi agreed to help Patti prepare for a special visitor—her former boyfriend, Chris #2. I helped bring the salon and spa to Patti's bedside by purchasing a dishwashing tub, a turkey baster, and two-gallon-sized plastic pitchers. In addition, I gathered several beach towels and plastic trash bags from home. Angi brought Patti's favorite Aveda hair supplies.

We arrived at 8:30 A.M., just as Patti was waking up. She had spent the night in her own bed, not the hospital bed in her living room; I was happy about that because nothing is better than your own bed. Carefully, we turned her backwards in bed and placed several pillows under her. This allowed her hair to fall back into the dishwashing tub. I brought Angi two pitchers of warm water and she went to work on Patti's hair. Meanwhile, David lit some candles and put on a CD with the sound of ocean waves. Patti's mom and I used some of the fancy lotions Patti had received as gifts and massaged her arms and hands and legs and feet. Her skin was as thin and delicate as tissue paper. After forty-five minutes of pampering, Patti needed a nap. As we left her apartment, she looked and smelled good, and was gently smiling as she fell asleep.

The best gifts are time and attention, not material things. Each visit with Patti helped me rediscover what was so easy to forget in my busy life. Although I would have preferred to rediscover these lessons another way, I was grateful for the reminder.

Thursday, Friday, and Saturday

After seeing Patti for three straight days on four separate visits, I began to feel guilty about spending so much "extra" time with her. Therefore, even though it was incredibly hard not to camp out by her bedside, I chose not to visit her on Thursday, Friday, or Saturday; that way, others could have an opportunity to spend time with her. I spoke frequently to Donna, though, and kept in close contact with Jen and Kim. My husband, Chris, and I planned to visit Patti on Sunday.

During my drives to and from Patti's apartment, I reflected on how to come to terms with what was happening. When Patti and I became "chemo friends" we were both in the infusion room at our oncology clinic, each receiving the same medication for treatment of our bone mets. We viewed our infusions as a mere inconvenience we were willing to live with so that we could do just that—live. It seemed unfair that Patti's cancer was so much more aggressive than mine; but her attitude and resolve were so positive that it never occurred to me that she would die from the same disease I had. Now it was happening, and only a few weeks after she had turned twenty-nine. I couldn't help reflecting that what was killing her could kill me, too. Breast cancer kills approximately forty thousand women each year. Suddenly, those statistics really hit home. Breast cancer kills.

My daily work seemed insignificant compared to this final stage of Patti's life. I was assisting with the launch of a new clinical drug study and was supposed to be planning an important meeting in Dallas, but when I told my boss about my friend, she told me to spend whatever time I needed with Patti. My boss knew I was a worker-bee and that I would not compromise the quality of my work even though I was going through a difficult time. And I also knew that if I allowed that to happen, Patti would be mad at me: She had her own amazing work ethic, and she took pride in it.

Sunday

When Chris and I arrived at Patti's on Sunday, most of the visitors were Patti's coworkers. I was very restless during this visit. Many conversations were going on; most did not include Patti, who lay with her eyes closed most of the time. People talked about topics that had nothing to do with anything Patti cared about—or at least that was my perception. But when I complained to Chris later, he had a different take on the situation. Maybe Patti was happy just to hear the chatter and to know that her friends were near, he said. I had never considered that. But I did tell him that if I was ever in the same situation, we would need a code word I could use so that he would intervene if my visitors behaved that way. I think Chris thought I was nuts, but he went along with me—probably because he hated to hear me speak of my own possible death.

Though I was frustrated by the visit, it was good for Chris. He held Patti's hand, and when he asked permission to kiss her forehead, Patti opened her eyes and with a "knowing look" smiled and nodded. It created a good memory for Chris to hold on to.

Monday

I was scheduled to make a presentation at a Ribbons of Pink (ROP) event that evening. But on Monday morning, a severe migraine put me flat on my back. I think the migraine was my body's way of telling me to take it easy. I had been freaking out about what was happening to Patti and juggling my visits to her bedside with working extra long days to get ready for the Dallas meeting. And, in addition, there was my "second full-time job" as president of ROP.

I wondered, too, whether the migraine had showed up because I was afraid to get up in front of young women and teach them about early detection and breast health at the same time I knew Patti was dying. I tried to remind myself that early detection in Patti's case gave her several years of life she might otherwise not have had. Still, I was disheartened by the harsh reality that in the midst of our positive attitudes and our "We are breast cancer survivors, hear us roar!" mentality, breast cancer was killing my dear friend.

Tuesday and Wednesday

Again, I gave up my place on the visitors' list so that others could visit Patti. I was still recovering from my migraine and feeling worn out. Was I slowly withdrawing from Patti on a subconscious level to make the impending loss less painful?

Thursday

En route to the airport to fly to Dallas for the meeting I had helped plan, I stopped to see Patti. Her self-imposed two-week countdown was nearing its end. When I arrived, Patti was asleep, looking very weak. Her skin tone was more jaundiced (yellowing caused by liver failure), and her abdomen was filled with fluid. I held her hand, but she didn't stir until suddenly, without warning, she opened her eyes, smiled, and exclaimed, "I missed you!"

Whether she thought I was someone else or knew that it really was me I will never know, but I treasure the memory of that moment. I placed a flower behind her ear and told her it looked great. She smiled a sweet, peaceful smile and fell asleep again. I kissed her forehead and left. All the way to the airport, I cried. I knew this was probably my last visit with her, and it broke my heart. However, I had a business meeting to conduct, and to cancel it would have upset Patti, so I continued with my life just as hers was slipping away.

Friday

While I was out of town, Patti was constantly on my mind. When I called to check in during my breaks throughout the day and learned that her stream of visitors continued, I was relieved. I think she was trying to prove to her doctors that she could hang on for the full two weeks that she said she would.

Saturday

I had just returned to my hotel room after our final meeting when Chris called. Jen had phoned and told him that Patti died late that afternoon. With tears streaming down my face, I quickly hung up with Chris and called Jen. Even as I struggled to understand why Patti had to die, I pictured her in heaven: She'd made fifty new friends, had become godmother to many kitties and dogs, and was enjoying unlimited cherry limeades while relaxing with the fragrance of her favorite Yankee Candles.

Sunday

I flew home early the next day, and at noon, the FOP (Friends of Patti) gathered with her family to plan Patti's local memorial service. We convened at Donna's house. Patti's brother, David, took notes. I'm not sure I knew everyone who was there, but we were all in pain and all determined to make Patti's memorial service a meaningful one. We knew Patti would have crinkled her nose at the whole thing, but we hoped she would understand that the FOP needed to say good-bye and have closure with her death.

Everyone agreed the service should include some of Patti's favorite music, especially songs from the contemporary church services she attended—"Rock & Roll Church" as she called it. We picked songs. Scriptures. And a poem she liked. An excerpt of her writing from this book was also included, as well as an excerpt from her Alpha Sigma Alpha (ASA) sorority creed. We agreed to put up a "memory board" where people could tack their favorite personal photos of Patti. And we planned to honor Patti's "God-animals." Patti was the godmother to so many dogs (and two cats—mine). She loved them all dearly, and they loved her. Finally, in lieu of punch or coffee and tea, we agreed to serve Patti's favorite cherry limeade. Donna offered to secure the ingredients so that they would be the real thing.

Saturday

At Patti's local memorial service, the minister who spoke about Patti mentioned that in a church of more than ten thousand members, she had not known that Patti was a young breast cancer survivor or patient. And then she explained that this was because Patti had deliberately decided that church would be the one place where no one would know. It was the one place where she could be normal and not labeled "sick."

Driving home with Chris after the service, I reflected again on Patti's life, and how she had made a difference to me and my world. She helped me overcome my fear to live and helped me not be afraid to die. She taught me how to swim. She showed me that sometimes pushing the limits of our bodies is necessary to help boost our mental and physical confidence. She trusted her doctors and knew that medical treatments could help prolong her life, but she realized that God is the one in control. She lived her life as she wanted—not as others thought she should—and she lived with purpose. Patti was, and will always be, my inspiration.

I knew all along that Patti's situation was serious, but she hid it well. To look at her physically fit body and full head of hair, you would have no idea that she was a Stage IV breast cancer patient who had somehow managed to live past the standard two-year survival rate. Yes, the cancer had spread to her liver, lungs, and bones, but she lived her life in spite of these circumstances.

Patti was so busy socially that we had to schedule time with her well in advance. What with softball games, travels, Bible study nights, singles activities at church and work, she was going a hundred miles an hour.

In November of the prior year, 2002, we knew her health had taken a slide. She stopped her maintenance chemotherapy for a few weeks so that she could receive radiation to her back for bone mets pain. You can't have chemotherapy and radiation at the same time, but stopping the chemo let the cancer grow like a wildfire.

Looking back, I see it all so clearly. I feel foolish for not recognizing that my friend was slowly dying. In January, she vomited so violently that she broke a few ribs. Despite our urging her to stay home and rest, she went to Las Vegas as she had planned. Perhaps she knew it would be her last chance to take a fun trip with a friend.

In February, her abdomen started filling with fluid because the cancer had grown so large that it impaired her liver function. She must have known her body was shutting down, but she didn't tell us. She invited her mom to come to one of our luncheons while she was in town. She even brought a camera to take pictures. I realize now that Patti was preparing for the end of her life.

We celebrated Patti's twenty-ninth birthday at our last "official" book writing meeting on March 8. I joked with her in my birthday card that she'd better look out for next year because we were going to tease her about turning thirty. I wanted so much to believe she would make it to her thirtieth birthday!

Patti literally willed herself to drive over to that book meeting held at Jana's house, but she slept through most of it due to her pain medication. Jana, Kim, and I were worried, but we still didn't acknowledge that the end was so near. And every so often, when we got stuck on how to word something in our outline, Patti gave us hope by chiming in with a great idea. However, we did talk her into letting Kim drive her home.

When Patti was admitted to the hospital for dehydration and to have her abdomen drained again, her friend Donna kept us in the loop, but said the family didn't want any visitors that weekend. We didn't know it then, but her oncologist had privately told her family that it could be a matter of days before Patti passed away.

Now that I am a parent, I can't imagine hearing the words "We are out of options." How do you deal with something like that? Patti knew she was very, very ill, but with her usual verve and drive, she set her own timeline: two weeks. She had two weeks to live.

When Jana called to tell me of her conversation with Patti— and Patti's "two weeks"—I went numb. I kept thinking that something could be done. This vibrant woman had played softball the summer before. She'd been active in breast cancer events in October. This was Tigger, who bounced back from everything. What were the doctors missing?

I sent an e-mail to everyone I knew, asking for their prayers. I was reaching for a miracle—one that I knew was not likely, but I hoped for it nonetheless.

I was six weeks from my baby's due date, so Matt tried to keep me calm, but I couldn't stop crying. My heart hurt so much! I had lost several grandparents, and that was painful, but they were older. Their passing was more expected.

In the two years that I'd known Patti, I had grown to love her as a sister. She was so young! It seemed unfair that I'd been given the chance to have two children, but Patti would never know the joy of motherhood.

Jana, Kim, and I met at Nordie's the next day to regroup. We were painfully aware that all four of us would never sit together again. We needed to find out whether Patti wanted us to continue the book project even if she passed away. The book had been so important to her. She had already written many of her chapters, and she had tons of journal entries about her breast cancer experience. It would be hard, but if she wanted us to finish it, we would.

When I returned to work after lunch, I couldn't concentrate. Jana called and said we'd been given the green light to visit Patti in the hospital. Patti's mom and dad and her brother, David, were there, too. Patti adored David. None of us had met her dad before that day, but he and the whole family were calm and gracious. I was a nervous wreck.

Patti looked so frail and tired, and her tummy was hugely distended from the fluid. I was eight months pregnant, and, true to form, Patti managed a whispery joke about knowing how I felt. We were not sure how to broach the subject of the book, and we were relieved when she did it for us. She told us that the book was important and she wanted us to complete it. Her unspoken message was, "Even if I'm gone."

I went home and cried. Parker hugged me and tried to make me feel better, and as I wrapped my arms around my little boy, I hurt again for Patti's parents because they were losing their beloved child.

She had bought a new SUV six months earlier. She had even signed a five-year loan: "Hey, I'm going to be around," she said. She planned to adopt two little Chinese girls whether or not she found the man of her dreams. How could Patti be at the end of her life?

I had an appointment the next day with my obstetrician. I remembered Patti's excitement when she learned I was pregnant again. She was so happy that I was able to have a child after breast cancer. Now she would never meet my child.

Previously, Matt and I had decided to let our baby's sex be a surprise. Now I decided that the one gift I could give Patti was to let her know the sex of the baby. So my obstetrician scheduled an ultrasound, and we found out we were having a baby girl. Patti had been sure I was having a girl, so I knew this would thrill her.

On Tuesday, Patti was at home again, and Jana, Kim, and I went to see her. She looked much better. After we had asked the necessary questions for her portion of the book, I told her I had news. As soon as I said, "It's a girl," she commented, "I knew it! Now what are we going to name her?"

Her mom thought she was holding on to life for some reason, so we made it clear to Patti that we had everything we needed for the book. If she was ready, there was nothing stopping her.

I had my last visit with Patti a few days before she passed away. She was sleeping in the bed she loved. I think she recognized me. She talked a little, though her voice was very weak. I knew the end was not far off, and I held her hand tightly. I thought of a million things I could say to her; but my time was limited, and in the end, the most important thing to say was "I love you." I gave her a big hug and kissed her on the forehead. She was smiling and looked very peaceful.

A few days passed. I planned to see Patti on Saturday after we took Parker to a *Disney on Ice* production and to his friend's birthday party, but, before I knew it, the day had slipped away. When I called that evening to check on Patti, her mom answered. Patti had passed away half an hour before. Her sorority sister Dione was holding her hand when she died.

Though I knew it was coming, the actual words—the realization that she was gone!—left me stunned. I called Jana and Kim to let them know.

It was Patti's wish to be cremated, but not being able to view her body made it harder for me to come to grips with the reality that she had died. Seeing a body in a casket, as morbid as it might seem, brings a sense of finality for me.

In our original book outline, we didn't have a chapter on death and dying, but now it became a chapter we had to write. It's still hard to understand why Patti had to leave us at such a young age. It seems so unfair. She caught her tumor as early as possible with self-exams. My comfort comes from knowing that Patti lived her short life to the fullest. She treated each day as a gift. She inspired others, and I'm sure she is now in heaven, acting as a greeter, making sure everyone else feels at home. Finishing this book without her has been hard, but I feel that she is guiding us in spirit.

Kim

Where do I begin? We all knew that Patti was a Stage IV cancer patient who had fought with everything she had for several years. But it was easy to forget how sick Patti was. She stayed as active and as positive as a perfectly healthy person. Patti made her full life look so easy. She inspired me and many others by refusing to let cancer stop her from living.

I was elected president of our college sorority the same year Patti pledged. Little did I know that she would follow in my footsteps as president, and that later, she would save my life. Two years after Patti's recurrence, I was diagnosed and I caught it early because I performed my monthly breast exams after hearing about Patti's experience. I always told Patti she was my guardian angel.

In October 2003, Patti presented me with the Ribbons of Pink "You Are an Inspiration" recognition, an honor she herself had received the previous year. In her speech, she said, "Kim, when I was diagnosed with breast cancer four years ago, I remember thinking that if I could make a difference in one person's life by helping her catch her cancer early enough, I could count my battle as one well fought. I never dreamed that person would be you."

From day one of my breast cancer diagnosis, Patti was there for me. I thought she would always be there, making us laugh with her uncanny humor and Patti-isms.

I guess I thought that if anyone could beat breast cancer, it would be Patti. But in November, things starting going downhill, and by February, fluid had built up in her abdomen. Because Patti was cramping a lot, her mom came to stay with her, and Patti brought her along to our February Nordie's lunch.

At our luncheon, Patti joked that her distended stomach was a sign of pregnancy, and the scary part was that she looked pregnant. Walking was hard for her, and she joked about being slower than her grandma. Despite her attempts to be light-hearted, she was not the bubbly, high-energy Patti we were used to. After lunch, Patti had her mom take a picture of the four of us. When I see the photo now, I can hardly believe how skinny and sick Patti looked. We were concerned after that lunch, but I still expected Patti to be her typical Tigger self and bounce back.

When Patti came to our last book-writing session in March, she was in no condition to drive, so I persuaded her to let me drive her home. On our way, I asked how she was really doing. She said she was tired, but that she was looking forward to getting back to work. She thought she might be promoted again and was excited about the possibility.

I wanted so hard to believe this would happen. But looking back, I wonder whether Patti already knew that she was nearing the end. Had the doctors told her something that we didn't know?

I felt such a sense of helplessness as I wondered what I could do. Knowing how much Patti enjoyed the spa, some of our sorority sisters and I planned a Patti Day at a local spa on March 29, free for cancer patients. Patti was excited about it.

By March 14, we learned that Patti was back in the hospital. I sent flowers and a card but I wanted to be there. Things were spinning out of control. I began to suspect the worst and yet—like Jen—part of me kept thinking: She's Tigger. She'll bounce back.

When Jen called to say Patti had only two weeks to live, I was astounded. I remembered how she had looked four months earlier when she presented me with the award at the Ribbons & Racquets gala. Her sexy sequined top and satin pants. She was so full of life! How could she now have just two weeks? As I sent e-mail updates to our sorority sisters, tears rolled down my face.

When I was diagnosed with breast cancer, I never asked, "Why me?" But now I asked, "Why Patti?" I almost felt it should be me instead of Patti. If it weren't for her, I wouldn't even be here because I wouldn't have discovered my lump. In one of Patti's journals, she said that all she wanted was to make it to her thirtieth birthday. That night, I got on my knees and prayed for a miracle. "Please, let her make it to thirty." I sent e-mails to everyone I knew, asking them to pray for Patti.

I also knew that many of my friends and family who didn't know Patti were praying for her, and were also thinking that this could be me. After all, I had the same type of cancer and had undergone the same treatment as Patti. Hers came back; so could mine. She was going to die; so could I.

Thinking about me even for a brief second left me feeling guilty. Patti needed me. I couldn't be worried about my own life. But I was angry and I let God know. Patti had done everything correctly, but her story wasn't ending as it should. She had saved my life; why couldn't I do something to save hers?

Jen's call that we should get to the hospital as soon as we could scared me. On the way, I picked up the inscribed picture frame we'd decided to give Patti, grateful that it was finished. Jana brought a copy of the picture, and we met at the hospital an hour later. One of my sorority sisters had dropped off a basket of goodies that we prepared for Patti—Yankee Candle ocean breeze scent, a CD of the sound of ocean waves, flowers, lotion, and a blanket. Although I hoped Patti would enjoy everything, right now "things" seemed immaterial.

In the hospital bed, Patti looked very frail. Her skin was a gray-greenish color. I instantly knew why we had received the call to come to the hospital. She didn't look as if she could make it for two more weeks. Yet in true Patti form, she insisted that she had lots to do. And she still wanted to prove the doctors wrong.

My grandfather had passed away, but I had never really known anyone else who had died. What should I say? How coherent would Patti be? These thoughts crossed my mind as I was driving to Patti's apartment for our scheduled visit on Tuesday. Her brother David greeted us, and I was struck by a strong fragrance of candles and flowers. Patti looked like a different person. Her color was back, and she was coherent, even able to joke with us. I felt my hope renew—maybe our prayers had been answered. We interviewed Patti for the book and massaged her hands and feet.

That night, Patti gave me a gift—the gift of peace. During our interview, we asked what advice she would give others in her situation. She said, "Give it up to God." Patti was not scared; she was at peace. As I left the apartment, I knew that Patti was going to die, but I also knew that she was going to be our angel in heaven. I did have one request, though. "Please, God, don't let Patti die on my birthday." If she did, I would feel as though God were taking her life to save mine. I know it sounds crazy and maybe selfish, but that night, I prayed to God, "Please give Patti her full two weeks."

I turned thirty-two on March 19 and wished I could give Patti one of my years so that she could be thirty. I didn't feel like celebrating. We went to visit Patti. Chris #2 was still with her, feeding her nectarines, which she loved, so instead we talked to Patti's mom. It seemed surreal when she began asking about ideas for Patti's memorial service. How could we be talking about a service when Patti was still alive, and in the next room?

The mail carrier brought mail as we sat there. He couldn't fit the seventy-five cards into the slot, so he had to ring the doorbell.

Strangely, at this time I felt a tremendous outpouring of support for me from my family and friends. I was surprised and even a little annoyed. After all, I wasn't the one who was dying. Patti was. They needed to be concerned about her and not worry about how I was holding up. Looking back, I know they prayed for Patti, but they were also concerned about my health.

On the day of the planned special spa event, the sorority sisters involved decided we should still get together and do something even though Patti couldn't be with us, so we went to a pottery store and painted our own pottery. I'm not at all artistic, but it felt therapeutic to paint and be surrounded by friends. I chose to paint a plate. I drew a pink ribbon in the middle and wrote "Nordie's at Noon" below. On the back, I put the date, March 29, 2003, and our names—Jana, Jen, Kim, and Patti. Ironically, this was the very day that Patti died. The Nordie's plate will forever be a special memory of Patti.

Sunday, Patti's family invited a few FOPs (Friends of Patti) to help plan the local memorial service. It was such a privilege to be included. We all had stories of Patti, most of them told with much affectionate laughter. Patti's parents planned to have a separate memorial service in her hometown. Our cele-bration of Patti's life would reflect her life and personality.

I stayed busy over the next week, preparing inserts for our Celebration of Life program. They included a "Memories of Patti" section, our sorority creed, and an excerpt from *Nordie's at Noon*. It helped me to feel I was contributing something, and it kept my mind off the fact that she was no longer with us.

Before Patti's memorial service on Saturday, I met with soror-ity sisters who were also Patti's friends. We toasted Patti's life with margaritas, knowing this is how she would have wanted it. The service was difficult and beautiful, all at the same time.

The very next day, Scott and I left for Florida for a vacation we had planned several months previously. This was our first vacation since I was diagnosed with breast cancer. On the beach in Marco Island, we spelled Patti's name in the sand and toasted her with champagne at sunset. I could feel Patti's presence watching over us.

Although I am at peace with Patti's death, it doesn't make me miss her any less. She helped me realize that we should live life to the fullest while we're here so that when it's our time, we can give it up to God and be at peace. What an amazing insight

from a twenty-nine-year-old woman who knew she was going to
die. I thank Patti's spirit every day for teaching me wonderful
lessons—about living, about dying, about hope.

Patti

I wanted to be the one to put the finishing touches on this
chapter. I wrote most of what you'll read, but I didn't finish
this chapter alone. My mother, father, and brother finished it
for me, and to them I am grateful. Below are the choices I
made during my second bout with cancer and a sense of how
those choices sustained me.

The Choice to Live and Not Be Afraid to Die

This is actually a two-part lesson. The first part, I noted in
chapter 3. For many people, making the choice to "live" (a.k.a.
"beat the cancer") comes at some point after the initial diagnosis. I ended the chapter with "Cancer wasn't going to beat me; I
was up at the line again."

The choice to live without being afraid to die didn't come
until two years later when I learned my breast cancer had
metastasized. In retrospect, that's sad to me, because it was actually the greater of the two-part lesson to learn. Willing yourself to live often takes sheer guts and a willingness to do "what
it takes" to reach a goal. Living without being afraid to die
takes being at peace with where you are in life. That peace
wasn't a part of my Peter Pan-ish, twenty-four-year-old self. It
takes a lot of looking within yourself, looking back at your life
and answering certain questions: Have I done everything I set

out to do here on earth? Am I right with everyone that I've wronged? Am I happy with my spiritual relationship with God? Am I living without regrets?

I wasn't able to answer yes to any of those questions when I was initially diagnosed. However, by the second time around, I'd managed to answer yes to every one of them. It gave me a great feeling of peace to be ready to die. It finally allowed me to "live" in some ways. I became much more free with my emotions and willing to take chances that I would not have taken before. Maybe I didn't take those chances in the past because I was afraid, or maybe because there was no impending "death" looming over me to make me understand that "tomorrow might be too late." The second time around, I learned not to wait for important things.

Jana said that having cancer gives you a sense of "urgency" that others do not experience. As you find you are no longer afraid to die, I think it manifests within you a very real sense of what it is to "live," and what it takes to do so. It was a wonderful moment of clarity and freedom to realize I'd finally made the impact on earth that I wanted. I found that I spent my days living as though they were gifts, or freebies. Picture me saying, each day as I wake up, "No whammies, no whammies, Patti wants another day to 'make a difference,'" and you'll understand.

It's certainly more freeing than waking up being afraid that this is your last day on earth and not being at peace with what you've done with your time here. I highly recommend this stage of living, but caution you to take your own time getting there. If you wonder why, please refer to the "best advice that Patti ever got" about living cancer as one's own individual experience (chapter 3). You can't force losing your fear of death; you can only begin to ask yourself the questions that will lead you there.

The Choice to Make a Difference

I believe that choosing to "make a difference" is a crucial part of reaching that Zen-like existence where you're not afraid to die. I think it is human nature to want to make a difference.

So how do you go about it? Well, it's as individual as each person and her cancer experience. After my first chemo experience, I chose to challenge my body to become a machine of sorts. I started running short road races, and I completed my first triathlon. I wanted to celebrate the body that had survived this nasty, horrible disease, and challenging my body athletically was one way I could do that.

I became an advisor to a nearby chapter of my national social sorority. Each time I spent an evening working with these wonderful, talented women, I knew it was one of the best things I could do with my time . . . hands down! In one evening a month, I was able to "make a difference" in seventy women's lives.

I started taking my philanthropic work in the community more seriously. I began to tithe to my church. I was elected to the board of directors for the Ribbons of Pink Foundation. I wanted to become a champion for breast cancer, but at the same time have a life that did not focus totally on breast cancer. I started to seek balance.

I made my work become a meaningful part of my existence instead of letting it be just a "job." This choice led me to produce some of my best work because I chose to care about what I was doing.

I allowed myself to care about people, too, without judging or having unfair expectations; to love them unconditionally. I think I fell in love for the first time when I made that choice. It was both heart-breaking and uplifting. Before choosing to make a difference, I never would have had the chance to experience the sense of joy with which I now live.

I gave myself unselfishly, and the outcome was more happiness. I did things "in an effort to glorify God," and that sense of greater purpose helped me find energy to do all the things I had to do most days.

In choosing to "make a difference" through touching other people's lives, I found true happiness within my own. Curious how that works, isn't it?

The Choice to Come Out of Cancer a Better Person

You could spend the rest of your life asking: "Why? Why me? Why now?" But I counter, "Why not? Why not me? Why not now?"

There is no rhyme or reason to why you get cancer. No one promises you the answer; no one even promises that you'll live. (Thankfully, with advances in screening and treatment, this is becoming more and more an option.) No one promises that you'll look good with no hair, but I think you'll be pleasantly surprised by how many people do look good bald. You have a choice about how you want to deal with cancer because, even as the disease takes control of your body, you do still have control over certain things.

You can control that you get out of bed with a smile on your face. You can treat each day like the gift that it is. If you have mastered the "nonfear of death," this should be second nature to you. You can come out of cancer a healthier person. You can choose to make the most of what time you do have here on earth.

You can walk through cancer and become a more emotive, loving person. Before these last two years, I was restrained, fearing to open myself up to others. I was afraid to write a book—or even a chapter—about how cancer made me feel and how I reacted to it. After all, I thought, people I will never meet will read this book. At one time, a willingness to open my heart to them was a scary proposition. But you can choose to overcome that fear. You can choose so much about cancer, even as it seems to take choices away from you.

I learned that I had Stage IV breast cancer in September 2000. A lot of what happened after that is shared in this book. I made the choices above during my recurrence. They renewed the gift of life in me and sustained me during my last two weeks.

In February 2003, my liver began to fail. I was in and out of the hospital over the next month and, in mid-March, I returned home for Hospice care. Before I left the hospital, I spoke with my doctors. They said, "We'd love to see you prove us wrong this time. We really, really would." "But based on my test results?" I asked, and they said, "No." My surgeon cried. Later, my oncologist took my hand and said, "I've done everything I can do." I answered, "It's okay."

You have to believe in the power of faith and give it up to God.

And I did.

I left the hospital and returned home. The Nordie Girls came to see me; Donna and Dione were there and I loved them; Chris drove up from Dallas, and my brother made chocolate shakes (I think he kept slipping in some Ensure!). We lit candles and received flowers. When the mail came, I exclaimed, "Oh, my! More letters," and then listened as my dad read them aloud to me. We played good music. My coworkers, sorority sisters, friends, and family from near and far stopped by. My massage therapist and my mother gave me massages. My brother brought me a plastic goose for a nightlight; I named it Gander. There were some less nice moments; but mostly I wanted to be like a sponge and soak it all up. I wanted to soak it all up so I could keep it with me.

And I did.

CHAPTER ELEVEN

Life Is Still Good!

— Nordie's Café —
April 2005

Jen and Kim eagerly waited for Jana to arrive at their corner booth at Nordie's. This was a special day. Jana was coming from San Francisco, where she had moved a year earlier. She was in town because this Nordie's lunch marked the second anniversary of Patti's death. It was important for everyone to be together to reflect on Patti's life and share the experiences of the past two years.

Jana arrived and hugs ensued. The Nordie Girls were together again. As everyone settled in, Jana picked up her glass to give a toast. "Here's to Patti Sue, who is enjoying her chocolate mousse cake in heaven. Here's to us as we continue to celebrate life and try to live our lives as Patti did." We clinked our glasses of water, iced tea, and soda together. "Here's to Patti and to us," we repeated, with smiles on our faces.

"Life is good" was Jana's mantra during her first cancer diagnosis, and the motto was adopted by all of us. In spite of the group's collectively having had sixty rounds of chemotherapy, more than fifty radiation treatments, six mastectomies, two breast reconstructions, four breast implants, four recurrences, one diagnosis of lymphedema, and too-numerous-to-count medical tests, including bone scans, CT scans, MRIs, mammograms, ultrasounds, and blood draws, since our cancer journeys began, the sharing of experiences enabled us to meet at Nordie's, where we were now toasting Patti and reflecting, with smiles: "Life is still good!"

Monthly luncheons at Nordie's had provided a forum for deep friendships to develop, for fears to be expressed and understood, and for mutual support to be offered. The normalcy of the routine and pleasant surroundings of the café provided comfort even during the most stressful and unnatural time of all— the days leading up to Patti's death.

After losing a dear friend and coauthor, we vowed to remember Patti's greatest lesson: "Live life to the fullest and receive each day as a gift." As a result of breast cancer, every one of us— Jana, Jen and Kim—chose to live each day in gratitude; we chose to enjoy sunsets more often, to eat dessert first, or simply to say "I love you" more often.

Friendships that began with the words "You have breast cancer" blossomed into something deeper that defines a part of each "Nordie Girl" as well as our honorary "younger brother," David. We look forward to meeting at Nordie's again for many years to come. And although there are no guarantees in life, we'll take each day as the gift it is and always appreciate that life is still good.

Patti

I liked taking road trips. Traveling down a road in my car on a sunny day to any destination, planned or not, was one of my favorite things to do. I liked visiting friends. Celebrating a wedding. Or just getting the heck out of Dodge.

I loved looking at my kitchen wall, which was covered with pictures of friends, babies, and me—"the pet godmother"— hugging and spoiling my friends' cats and dogs.

I liked Adam Sandler, Julia Roberts, and Eddie Murphy movies. *Sex and the City* could always be counted on for a good laugh on a down day. I enjoyed sitting courtside at KU (University of Kansas) basketball games (though secretly I still liked Duke).

I didn't get to say these things in the previous chapters. They weren't really a part of "my cancer experience." Instead they were part of who I was in a life that was larger than cancer, but irrevocably altered by it.

A good moment came in August 2001 at a breast cancer event I attended. Ribbons & Racquets is a gala/auction that benefits the Ribbons of Pink Foundation. At the event, I received the "You Are an Inspiration" recognition. But that's not the kicker. In the audience, I spied a great-looking couple. "They look a lot like my mom and dad," I thought. Thirty seconds later, I said to myself, "Those *are* my parents." They had come to surprise me and watch me accept my award.

During the presentation, the speaker pulled quotes about me from my friends, family, and medical team. Then she did a far sneakier thing: She pulled quotes right out of my journal entries in which I had expressed my hopes and fears associated with cancer. I have to admit I got a little teary and felt a big warm fuzzy. It felt better than being named sorority sweetheart, getting my first real job, or being told that I was loved by a boy I loved back.

I think that's because facing cancer was the hardest thing I ever did. Harder than preparing corporate training classes. Harder than finishing the triathlon. Harder than having my heart broken.

As I listened to the presenter sharing my own words and the words of friends and family, I thought, "That person they're talking about really has worked hard, done good things, touched lives. And she did it without any hair, with limited energy, and sometimes on heart strength alone." I allowed myself a minute to be touched by the fact that I had kept on living, even when "the experts" said I should be dying.

Life was a little bit sweeter after that night.

After I died, those things were brought to mind again at a touching memorial service for me in Kansas City.

Another memorial service was held in my hometown of Farber, Missouri, where my dad is the minister and where the church breathes an emotion and spirit that can only be found in a small town. A good friend of the family, Rim Massey, preached. He said, "There is no fear in love, but perfect love casts out fear," and led the congregation in singing "Blest Be the Tie That Binds." Following the service, the women of the church and town provided a generous meal. And afterward, my ashes were buried at Mt. Olivet Presbyterian Church.

At both services, friends and family shared a favorite memory of me. This sharing created a beautiful reciprocity: The people who had nourished and enriched my life found my presence in their lives likewise nourishing and enriching, even after my death.

Friends shared memories such as:

"She never smiled halfway."

"I remember her humor and her courage in adversity."

"She embraced life joyfully."

"She was so upbeat and had such a positive attitude."

"When faced with a tough decision, I would often ask myself, 'What would Patti do?'" And,

"She made me forget she had cancer—maybe that's what she wanted."

Patti lives on in the hearts and lives of the people she touched and by generous contributions to the organizations and charities that were dear to her.

Jana

My surgeon warned me: "Cancer will not change you. It will amplify who you already were before you were diagnosed." So if you're a "glass-half-empty" person before cancer, you'll have a negative experience. But if you saw your world through rose-colored glasses before cancer, then you'll find some rose-tinged moments during and after your diagnosis.

I was viewing life through rose-colored glasses before my diagnosis. My career was developing in a field I loved. I was recently engaged. Quite simply, I was happy. My glass was half full then, and has only become more full during the experience. Let me explain.

At the time of this writing, I have lived for eight years since the fateful day I first felt the lemon-drop lump in my breast. During those years, I went through one lumpectomy and biopsy and was diagnosed with Stage I multifocal breast cancer. I had a mastectomy with no reconstruction, four rounds of high-dose chemotherapy, hair loss, two wigs, a fake boob, and a toxic, painful reaction to chemotherapy.

I also had one fabulous wedding and honeymoon, and I have celebrated seven wedding anniversaries since.

When cancer spread to my bones and I was diagnosed with Stage IV cancer, a drama-packed visit to the M. D. Anderson

Cancer Center brought me the disconcerting message that I had a 20 percent chance of surviving for five years. A Port-a-Cath was permanently inserted, and I began the first of what now totals more than sixty-two consecutive Aredia monthly infusions. Zoladex put me into premature menopause with thousands of hot flashes and forty pounds of weight gain. A prophylactic mastectomy prior to reconstructive surgery led to the discovery of more cancer in my chest-wall muscle. After thirty-three zaps of radiation, I completed my bilateral breast reconstruction with saline implants.

The reality that this disease can be fatal became undeniable after my dear "chemo friend" Patti died from it.

In the midst of all of these events, it would have been easy to become a glass-half-empty person. But my surgeon was right: Breast cancer amplified who I was prior to being diagnosed, which is why I can say that life is still good!

Foremost, it's because my faith has grown and I am finally beginning to understand my purpose in life. Simply, I am here to serve God. From Patti's writings, it's obvious that she lived her life to glorify God. I never fully understood it, though, until months after she was gone.

Now I wake up each morning realizing that this day is a gift and there are no promises for tomorrow. One day will be my last day, but even that day will be good because I believe I will be going somewhere even better.

Chris and I have packed more into our seven years of marriage than many couples do in their entire lifetimes. We have honeymooned in Maui, traveled extensively around the United States, gone on Caribbean cruises, swum with dolphins, vacationed in Oahu and Kauai, and bought a time-share in the desert. We built a new house in the suburbs, then quit our jobs in the Midwest and moved to San Francisco in pursuit of an action-packed life in a city I always dreamt of living in. And, we have two sweet cats who greet us when we come home each day. Each day, our love grows stronger. We have a solid relationship I never imagined possible.

In celebration of my fifth year of survival, I had a pink ribbon tattooed onto my ankle. My parents were shocked and disappointed. "Some day you'll regret it," they warned.

I hope I do live long enough to regret having a tattoo. Or maybe I will not regret it, and instead will be showing it off to my fellow gray-hairs at the retirement center when I am ninety. By then, it will look like a small blob on wrinkled skin, but I will proudly explain how, sixty-odd years earlier, it was a badge I wore to remind myself of what I had gone through. And that is what it is—a badge.

My surgical scars are also badges and reminders, but I don't often look at them any more, and they are even beginning to fade. My ankle tattoo is something I can easily glance at. It visibly reminds me that I must never take a day for granted. It reminds me that hope and faith carried me through one set of difficult times and will carry me through again when I need special strength and courage.

Today, I sometimes forget about the disease that could some day take my life. Of course, I think about it when I go for my monthly infusions and lab work. I think about it when I am lying on a CT scan table, hoping nothing is found. I think about it when I get my prescriptions refilled. But I no longer think about it every day.

To live my life as I believe God wants me to, I have created two lists. The first is what I absolutely must do before I die. The second is a list of what I want to do before I die. I may not make it all the way through the second list, but I'm going to try.

The first list is more difficult and holds challenges. It is, by far, more important. Some of the things I learned from Patti: "Living a life that glorifies God, making sure relationships in my life are right, and striving to fulfill my life's purpose."

The second list includes things such as my career aspirations and places I want to visit. It's much more "fun" and includes only things that really won't matter after I die.

I don't believe I went through all I have gone through to help just one person. I want to help as many people as possible. I hope to reach thousands of women and educate them about breast health. I want to help other young survivors. That's why I've spent countless hours working with several breast cancer organizations, including the one I founded in 1999, the Ribbons of Pink Foundation (ROP).

Inspiration for ROP came from two places. First, when I was diagnosed, there were no organizations that focused on young women with breast cancer. Second, fourteen months after my initial diagnosis, as I drove around an upscale shopping center, I saw brightly colored banners adorning each of the light posts around the parking lot. I had an idea. October is National Breast Cancer Awareness Month. Why not display giant pink ribbon banners on the light posts in October to promote breast cancer awareness?

After a few phone calls and meetings, the shopping center management agreed to fund half the banners if I could raise the rest of the money. With the help of my stepmom, we sold "advertising space" on specially designed tee shirts, and we raised several thousand dollars. We purchased banners, sold more tee shirts throughout October, and handed out breast cancer awareness information at tables set up in the shopping center. The remaining proceeds were donated to the American Cancer Society.

When I saw one hundred light posts, each alternating with a black or white background and a giant pink ribbon, I became teary eyed. The black banners were in memory of those who had died from breast cancer. The white banners represented hope and survivorship.

Soon the local media started interviewing me, and that gave me the idea of starting a nonprofit organization. The mission of ROP is to "Promote Breast Health & Support Young Breast Cancer Survivors." After more news stories, the ball began to roll, and it has continued to gain momentum. In 2005, ROP became a Fund of the Greater Kansas City Community Foundation and is no longer a free-standing organization. I am so proud that after many years of fund-raising efforts, ROP was able to set up a fund to provide grants to organizations that meet our mission for many years to come. This is a dream come true, and I am grateful to everyone who helped realize this dream. (For more information, visit www.ribbonsofpink.org.)

My involvement in ROP and other breast cancer organizations has made me aware of the importance of volunteering and donating financially to such charities. I also now make an effort to purchase items with pink ribbons that support breast cancer programs and research.

However, the simplest way I contribute to the breast cancer cause is by spending a few extra cents by mailing letters by using the Breast Cancer postage stamp. The multicolor stamp features the words "Fund the Fight" and "Find a Cure" and has raised several million dollars in the past eight years. The stamps were issued in the summer of 1998 as I was in the middle of my chemotherapy cycle, and preparing my wedding invitations. At that time, Chris and I felt it was important to use these stamps on everything, including our invitations, response cards, and thank-you notes. And we continue to use the stamps today. I am enthused that something as small as a postage stamp is making a major impact in the fight against breast cancer.

Having faced several disease recurrences, I am not certain anymore that I'm going to win this battle against cancer. But I am not going to stop fighting. I have accepted that I am not in control of the disease—but I am in control of how I choose to deal with it. So I will continue the prescribed medical regimens. I will choose to have a positive attitude. And I will choose to live each day as if it were my last, because it could be.

Jen

I could not imagine, on that cold November day when I first found my lump, that having cancer would end up being a positive experience. The lessons I learned will be with me for the rest of my life.

The first positive about my cancer is that, aside from being pregnant, I had a textbook case. My treatment had no complications. No delays. No issues. Over two years ago, I hit my five-year anniversary, the date when many would consider me "cured," and the further out I get, the lower the chance of recurrence. We cautiously, yet optimistically, celebrated this milestone.

From the beginning, I decided to fight with all my might and not feel sorry for myself. I chose the most aggressive treatment option possible. I chose to believe that God had a lot more work for me to do on this earth, the most important being to raise my children. I also accepted the possibility that I could die, so I made sure (and continue to make sure) that all my loved ones know how important they are to me.

The hill has been a tough climb. Instead of joyfully picking out nursery patterns while pregnant, I was wondering whether my unborn baby and I would make it, and whether I would be around to raise my child. Still, cancer has been a great teacher.

What have I learned?

I've learned that life is very precious. I try not to waste time on trivial affairs. I walk a fine line every day; this means balancing my desire to accomplish everything as I would if I didn't have a lot of time left, yet not focusing too much on "This could be my last time to do something."

I've learned that my babies have been given to me as special gifts to nurture and love while I am here. Occasionally, when I yearn for more peace and quiet, I remind myself that these two miracles were sent to help me through a hard time and to remind me that there is life after breast cancer. I look forward to being here for the big events in their lives, and time has helped me believe that I will be here.

I've learned to appreciate my amazing human body and the need to take care of it. I still love M&Ms or an occasional chip, but I now think about every bite I put into my body. I try to eat edamame (soy bean pods) for a snack instead of sweets or fats. Water or green tea has replaced soft drinks. And I want to pass on this lesson to both my children.

I've developed a deeper relationship with God, and I am growing spiritually. I fully relied on God to get me through this. There was just one set of footprints in the sand for a long time.

Now that I am healthy, it's easy to allow more distance to come between God and me, so I work at slowing down and feeling that closeness again.

I've learned to appreciate life's small moments. I'm better about keeping in touch with people, and I'm more open with my emotions so that those close to me will know how I feel.

The journey has not only taught me, it has taught those around me. It's made younger women I know become more aware of their bodies. They're less likely to let a doctor tell them they are "too young" so they "shouldn't worry" about a suspicious lump. Without facing the life-threatening illness themselves, my illness has helped them understand how short life is and how every day is worth rejoicing.

I've evaluated the things I did properly in my cancer treatment and the things I would change based on what I know now. I give this advice as a "breast cancer warrior," not a medical professional.

What did I do that was right?

I did my homework. I knew what questions to ask my doctors. I checked out the backgrounds of the doctors to whom I was referred. I owned my cancer experience. Because of my type-A personality, I did my own research. Others may want a family member to do it. Just as long as someone does research from reliable sources such as WebMD, the Susan G. Komen Breast Cancer Foundation, the American Cancer Society, or the Young Survival Coalition. Get second opinions when you are not comfortable with what a doctor has offered. Don't be afraid to ask why a particular course is being recommended. No one cares more about your course of treatment than you.

I was willing to receive the most aggressive treatment available. It meant having my breast removed and getting chemotherapy while pregnant, but I knew I needed to do those things. I met a woman who refused chemotherapy while she was pregnant because she wanted to wait until after her baby was born. By then, her cancer had spread, and she died before her baby's six-month birthday. Go for the gusto right from the beginning. Each case is different, so you must work with your medical team, but be willing to do whatever it takes to fight this thing.

During treatment, I listened to my body and I slowed down. I still worked, but I reduced my schedule as needed. And I tried to eat well. I believe these two factors enabled me to receive all my chemo treatments without delaying any. I wanted to finish my fight before my baby was born so that I could move on to raising my baby.

As hard as it was, I let people help me. This was a blessing for me and for them because friends and coworkers wanted to do something. Bringing food or running an errand allowed them to feel part of the team. They were able to participate in the experience. For me, all those delivered meals were a lifesaver. But don't be afraid to tell volunteers to bring you healthy food! During chemotherapy, sometimes there are things you just can't eat. Be honest with friends. They're putting in a lot of time and effort to prepare something. Make sure it's something you can eat.

I used laughter. Having one's body fail is a humbling experience. Being able to laugh at my situation helped. Making up a name for my breast form was only one of the ways. After my surgery, I also saw the humor in the mailings I began receiving from the American Association of Retired Persons (AARP). Since the average woman who gets breast cancer is in her sixties, apparently AARP got my name and assumed I was sixty. Matt and I still laugh when an AARP mailing shows up.

I also let the experience become a learning opportunity for my family, friends, and coworkers. I could have kept it all a secret, but I felt it was too important for people not to know. From the start, I wanted to educate other women. Somehow, I knew it would make a difference that I was willing to "go public." I forwarded advocacy e-mails, reminding friends to contact their senators for additional funding for cancer research. I sent friendly reminders to perform monthly breast self-exams. Advocacy is something I took on from day one.

At first, though, I gave myself time to be the patient. Only when I was ready did I become a source of support for others. At the beginning, my fears would probably have scared someone else. It took about a year and a half before I was at a place where I could help others. Then I became a volunteer for the Pregnant with Cancer Network and a Reach-to-Recovery volunteer for the American Cancer Society. I also talked to people who were referred to me by doctors or friends of friends.

I formed my own support group. The Nordie Girls are some of the few people on this earth who understand where I am coming from. Emotionally, our luncheons have been one of the best things for me. Anyone who is diagnosed should find the right support for her.

One of my favorite quotes is "That man is a success who has lived well, laughed often, and loved much" by Robert Louis Stevenson.

After I was diagnosed, I purchased a sign that hangs over my sink. It says, "Live Well. Laugh Often. Love Much." It reminds me to take care of myself, to love as deeply as I can, and to enjoy every moment.

Cancer also taught me to let loose a little. I was a person who believed the motto "Save your pennies for a rainy day." Now I take more chances. We bought a bigger house when I was only one year out from treatment. We began to travel more. Matt and I vacationed in Hawaii to celebrate our tenth wedding anniversary and my five-year milestone.

What would I do differently?

A few things. When my hair started thinning, I should have shaved it all off instead of watching each hair fall out of my head. If I did it again, I'd have a shaving/hat party at the first signs of losing my hair.

More pictures! I love pictures and scrap-booking, but I did not want pictures of myself bald. I have only one picture, taken with Parker, six weeks out of treatment when the fuzz was starting to show on my head. Now, I would like to reflect through pictures of all that I have been through.

I would have bought life insurance! Long before I became pregnant, I should have applied for a life insurance policy that was independent of the one my employer provided. Learning that insurance companies won't consider me a normal, healthy woman until I am cancer free for ten years was depressing. Now, although I like my career, I feel a bit trapped because my family can't afford for me to lose the life insurance provided by my employer. Luckily, my parents started a life insurance policy for me as a child that can be increased every three years without medical questions. It's not a big policy, but it is something. I have opened a policy like this for both of my children.

Breast self-exams beginning at age twenty can mean the difference between life and death. I am here because I found my lump just three months after a clinical exam. Get a baseline mammogram at age thirty-five (talk to your doctor if there is a family history) and have yearly mammograms starting at age forty. Have a yearly clinical breast exam by your physician along with a pelvic exam and a pap smear. Always remember: No one knows your body better than you.

Although I know this disease happens to younger women, I was floored when my pledge class sister, Julie (the one who asked me to whip out Boobsie at the lake), called me last summer to tell me that at age thirty-three, she too, had been diagnosed with breast cancer. I was thankful that I had been through this so that I could help her and let our friends know how to best support her. But I was angry that this disease had struck someone else I loved. It is for the Julies, Janas, Pattis, and Kims of the world, and for Emma's future, that I continue my fight against this disease.

I am so thankful that medical advances are being made every day. For instance, if I were diagnosed today, Herceptin would most likely be part of my first line of treatment options. In just a few short years, this significant research development has happened, and this leaves me hopeful. Researchers are also starting to find new ways to block the blood flow to tumors and prevent them from growing. I have so much hope that a cure for this disease will be found, and that Emma will live in a world where she does not have to live in fear of a breast cancer diagnosis.

Life is still good—in fact, it is more fulfilling than I could have ever imagined, and I would not erase my breast cancer experience from my life even if I could.

Kim

Many people who face a life-threatening disease will tell you later that it has changed their lives for the better. I am no exception. The lessons I learned by facing my own death from cancer, as well as from losing a dear friend and an aunt to the same disease, are lessons that most people don't learn until they're much older and wiser, if they learn them at all. I feel blessed to have such a great perspective on life at such a young age.

Breast cancer was the best teacher I ever had. After my diagnosis, I found strengths within that I didn't know I possessed. After hearing those fateful four words, "You have breast cancer," it was as if my entire life had flashed before my eyes. But not just the life I've already lived—also the life I was afraid I wouldn't be around to see. For me, surviving those private scary moments and being able to pull myself out of the depths of my own private hell made me a stronger person—a survivor! I made a conscious decision to go back to the doctor and fight this disease with all the strength I had. I chose to have all those surgeries and to put those poisonous drugs into my system to kill any stray cancer cells that might be floating around. I chose to concentrate on living, not the alternative. I looked at this journey as a major inconvenience in my life, and I tried to find the positive to help get me through.

Cancer taught me the importance of becoming an advocate; of asking the hard questions; of taking action and being proactive. I have learned it is important to be my own advocate and to take control of my own health and life. I realized that no one else was going to do it for me. I learned the importance of early detection—it saved my life. I learned to practice the three steps to breast health, namely, perform a monthly breast exam and get an annual clinical breast exam and an annual mammogram.

I made a list of questions and interviewed my doctors. I even took a tape recorder along. When one of my doctors did not answer my questions adequately, I got a second opinion and ended up changing doctors. Don't be afraid to get a second opinion and even a third opinion. It's your body and your life.

Cancer also taught me, as it did Jen, to accept help. This was a hard lesson because I'd always been the one giving help. But with no family in town, and my firefighter husband on twenty-four-hour shifts, I knew I couldn't keep up with our Energizer Bunny son while in chemotherapy. So I let my friends bring meals, baby-sit, and even clean my toilets. It helped them to know they were helping me.

This is what I tell people: "Hey, thanks to breast cancer, I got rid of my mommy fat with a tummy tuck, and I got a breast lift, too!" Humor is a healing factor. Precancer, I was uptight and serious; cancer taught me to laugh at myself and have more fun.

Prior to breast cancer, I was running the rat race, trying to be a super-mom, super-employee, super-aunt—trying to be just plain super. Looking back, I realize that I wasn't having much fun. I was so focused on my Palm Pilot that I forgot to enjoy life. Now I try to enjoy every minute. It's about making choices. Who cares if the house is a little dusty?

Before cancer, I had my life planned out—my five-year plan; my ten-year plan; my retirement plan. I had my entire life planned. Breast cancer taught me that, as John Lennon said, "Life is what happens while we're making other plans." We're not always in control.

The reality is that life is about uncertainty. But after a breast cancer diagnosis, it seemed that uncertainty was taking over my life. Those first few weeks of my diagnosis were very frustrating because I was not in control. For once in my life, I didn't have control over the situation. I couldn't put the bad days down in my Palm Pilot and schedule around them. Uncertainty seemed to surround me. I was uncertain about what the future held for me. However, none of us knows what the future holds, so we need to live for today. This wasn't an easy lesson to learn or to accept. I learned that life is precious and fragile and that you'd better make today count.

As a focused, driven person, precancer, I'd set a goal, reach it, and immediately move on to the next. Now my goal is to live a balanced life, which means spending time on things that are important—things I feel passionate about—and also leaving time to enjoy the unplanned moment.

For instance, one day as I was leaving a meeting, it started to rain. Other women were getting rides to their cars so that they wouldn't get wet, but I said, "No thanks." I walked to the car without an umbrella, enjoying the rain and not worrying about having a bad hair day.

I also learned to make time for myself—something that I didn't do enough of precancer. I read *People* and *US Weekly*; I get pedicures and manicures; I spend more time with family and friends; I travel more; I work less; and I say no more often.

Breast cancer gave me a newfound sense of freedom. I am not afraid of taking risks and of making mistakes. I've decided that I don't want to look back on my life when I'm eighty and, instead of seeing all the risks I took and goals I achieved, see excuses and reasons why I didn't try. I don't want to have any regrets. Life is too short.

Two years after my diagnosis, I realized that I had to follow my own advice. So I quit my high-paying law firm job to follow my passion. Since I was the chief breadwinner in our family (as I mentioned in an earlier chapter, my husband followed his own passion and hung up his business suit for a firefighter's suit), this decision carried some risk. However, it was a risk that I was willing to take. That's because cancer taught me to be less afraid of taking risks or of making mistakes. I am now making a difference, having fun, spending more time with family and friends, and earning a living at the same time.

As it did for the other Nordie Girls, breast cancer renewed my faith in God. My faith has been strengthened and I am now living each day as God's servant. Cancer helped me to see the big picture and realize that "the purpose of life is a life of purpose" (Robert Byrne).

Breast cancer reiterated to me that one person can make a difference. Although my parents taught me from an early age to give back to the community, my passion is even more focused as a result of my breast cancer. October, National Breast Cancer Awareness Month, will be filled with cancer awareness events for the rest of my life. I've had the honor through my breast cancer work to share the stage with governors, Miss America, and movie stars. For my advocacy efforts, I've been recognized nationally by Lifetime Television, *Self* magazine, and the Komen Foundation. However, for me, the most rewarding part has been helping other women when they're diagnosed with breast cancer. Through my "missionary" work of supporting newly diagnosed breast cancer patients and working with the Susan G. Komen Breast Cancer Foundation, the Young Survival Coalition, the American Cancer Society, the National Patient Advocate Foundation, and the many other great organizations for which I volunteer, I feel that I am making a difference. Margaret Mead said, "Never doubt that a small group of thoughtful committed citizens can change the world. Indeed, it is the only thing that ever has." Amen to that.

My breast cancer diagnosis also made me become even more of an advocate, not just with breast cancer patients, but with policymakers. Although I had been involved with politics all my life, it was after my breast cancer diagnosis that I realized the true value of public policy and advocacy. The reality is that politics affects every one of us every day. As a person living with breast cancer, I understand that reality now more than ever. Breast cancer. It's a health issue, a family issue, a women's issue, and, yes, breast cancer is a political issue. Why?

Because every day elected officials and other key policymakers make decisions about breast health and breast cancer care. Every day, politicians make important decisions about how much funding will be devoted to breast cancer research and who will have access to quality cancer care. These are not theoretical decisions. Breast cancer policies debated at the federal, state, and local levels affect everyone. This realization has made me become even more of an advocate for breast cancer research, education, screening, and treatment, from the halls of Congress to the White House, by getting involved with important public policy issues. I was very excited to be able to lead the Komen Champions for the Cure™ program for the Komen Kansas City Affiliate, and was even more honored when I was asked to join Komen's National Public Policy Advisory Council. Through these efforts, I feel I am using my talents and passion to help others. Each of us has a unique opportunity to become involved in public policy and shape not only the present but also the future. This ensures that those who come after us will be given the access and treatment they deserve.

For me, life is still amazingly good. I am living for the moment because tomorrow is never promised. I am not only surviving; I'm thriving. Along with Jana and Jen, and in memory of Patti, I hope that by sharing our stories, others will realize that life can still be good after breast cancer.

The Best Day of My Life

Today, when I awoke, I suddenly realized that this is the
best day of my life, ever! There were times when I wondered if
I would make it to today; but I did! And because I did
I'm going to celebrate!

Today, I'm going to celebrate what an unbelievable life
I have had so far: the accomplishments, the many blessings,
and, yes, even the hardships because they have served to
make me stronger.

I will go through this day with my head held high,
and a happy heart.

I will marvel at God's seemingly simple gifts:
the morning dew, the sun, the clouds, the trees, the flowers,
the birds. Today, none of these miraculous creations
will escape my notice.

Today, I will share my excitement for life with other people.
I'll make someone smile. I'll go out of my way to perform an
unexpected act of kindness for someone I don't even know.

Today, I'll give a sincere compliment to someone who
seems down. I'll tell a child how special he is,
and I'll tell someone I love just how deeply I care for them
and how much they mean to me.

*Today is the day I quit worrying about what I don't have
and start being grateful for all the wonderful things
God has already given me.*

*I'll remember that to worry is just a waste of time
because my faith in God and his Divine Plan ensures
everything will be just fine.*

*Tonight, before I go to bed, I'll go outside and raise my eyes
to the heavens. I will stand in awe at the beauty of the stars and
the moon, and I will praise God for these magnificent treasures.*

*As the day ends and I lay my head down on my pillow,
I will thank the Almighty for the best day of my life. And I
will sleep the sleep of a contented child, excited with expectation
because I know tomorrow is going to be . . .*

The Best Day of My Life!

GREGORY M. LOUSIGNONT, PH.D.

Postscript

In late November 2006, we headed to San Francisco to visit Jana and her husband, Chris, to celebrate the national book launch and to spend time together. At this time, Jana's cancer had spread to some of her organs and her mobility was limited. Though Jana was not able to show us around her beloved city by the bay, she had strict sightseeing orders for Kim, Jen, and Patti's brother, David. Popovers with strawberry butter at the Neiman Marcus Rotunda, a nightcap at The View atop the Marriott, and many other touristy attractions. And we had to document it all with pictures.

This trip would prove to be an important one for the Nordie girls and guys. A time for remembering. A time for celebrating. And a time for closure. Just two weeks after our visit, Jana's eight-year battle against breast cancer ended. Our hearts were broken, again, but through our faith we knew she was in a better place, without pain.

The passing of two of our co-authors has left an indelible mark on our lives, but more importantly, the lives they lived were examples of how to enjoy each day to the fullest and to make a difference in the short time we have here on earth. Their legacy lives on through the book and the many lives they continue to touch.

Since the release of *Nordie's at Noon* in 2006, we have been amazed at how our stories have impacted others. From the weekly e-mails we receive from readers and the feedback we hear as we travel the country sharing our message, *Nordie's at Noon* seems to give others hope and encouragement. We hope it is making the difficult journey that we all face after a cancer diagnosis a little bit easier. This was, and still is, our vision for *Nordie's at Noon*.

We have also been humbled by the recognition that our book has received. We are convinced Patti and Jana are up in Heaven orchestrating all of this as they have their own Nordie's lunches there. We were so proud in May, 2007 to receive the Natalie Davis Spingarn Writer's Award from the National Coalition of Cancer Survivorship. We were even more honored that our award was presented to us by Elizabeth Edwards, whose courage and grace continue to be an inspiration to all of us.

Who would have thought when we started meeting five years ago at Nordie's that we would now be touching so many lives? Kim and Jen carry on the Nordie's mission—educating others about early detection and supporting other survivors. Just as important, we continue raising money for and fighting against this disease until there is a cure.

There is a quote that fits Jana and Patti's enthusiastic approach to life that makes us smile when we think of them.

> *"Life should NOT be a journey to the grave*
> *with the intention of arriving safely*
> *in an attractive and well preserved body,*
> *but rather to skid in sideways, chocolate in one hand,*
> *wine in the other, body thoroughly used up,*
> *totally worn out and screaming*
> *"WOO HOO what a ride!"*

AUTHOR UNKNOWN

What a ride it has been.

Glossary

Adrenal gland: Gland found above each kidney that secretes steroid hormones, adrenaline, and noradrenalin.

Adriamycin (generic name, doxorubicin): A chemotherapy drug commonly used to treat breast cancer and other cancers. Adriamycin first disrupts, and then destroys, the growth of cancer cells.

Anesthesia: Loss of normal sensation or feeling. Certain drugs are used to produce anesthesia effects during surgery.

Aredia (generic name, pamidronate disodium): A medication that is used to reduce bone complications and bone pain in patients whose breast cancer has spread to the bone.

Areola (singular), areoles (plural): The circular field of dark skin surrounding the nipple.

Aromatase inhibitors: A class of drugs that block the production of estrogen from androgens, which are hormones in the body.

Autoimmune response: A condition in which the immune system attacks body tissues.

Bacterial endocarditis: An infection in the heart that is caused by the direct invasion of bacteria.

Barium: A compound used as contrast medium to enhance images for x-rays and CT scans.

Benign: Harmless; not cancerous.

Bilateral reconstruction: Surgery to rebuild the breast's shape after a mastectomy on the left and right sides.

Biopsy: Removing cells or tissues to identify disease. There are three types of biopsies:

1. Incisional or core: A sample of tissue is removed.
2. Needle or fine needle-aspiration: A sample of tissue or fluid is removed with a needle.
3. Excisional: A whole tumor or lesion is removed.

Bisphosphonate: A class of drugs used to strengthen the bones; these are administered intravenously.

Bone scan: A radiologic scan of the skeleton often used to detect bone metastasis.

Breast cancer staging: When a breast cancer diagnosis is made, a stage is assigned to aid in selecting the appropriate course of treatment and determining the prognosis. There are four primary stages (I, II, III and IV) and subcategories for different situations (e.g., Stage IIb). In determining the stage, several factors are taken into account, typically by using the TNM model. T is the tumor size, N is whether or not the cancer has spread to nearby lymph nodes, and M is whether or not the cancer has metastasized. Numbers or letters listed after the TNM provide more details about the cancer. The higher the stage number (e.g., Stage IV), the more advanced the cancer is. For more information about staging, visit www.cancer.org or www.komen.org.

Breast implant: A soft packet filled with silicone or saline that is inserted under the skin (and often the chest-wall muscle) to replace or enhance breast tissue.

Breast prosthesis: An artificial breast form that can be worn in the bra after a mastectomy. The prosthesis is typically made of silicone gel, fiber fill, or other materials that "feel" similar to real breast tissue.

Breast self-exam (BSE): A self-performed screening method that is intended to find tumors in the breast.

Cancer: A general term for more than one hundred diseases that are characterized by uncontrolled, abnormal growth of cells.

Chemotherapy: The term for the administration of medications used to kill cells that are rapidly reproducing. Both cancerous (unhealthy) and noncancerous (healthy) cells are affected by these drugs. There is also a type of chemotherapy that is called "targeted therapy." These drugs are less toxic to healthy cells, targeting only the cancer cells.

Clinical breast exam: A breast exam that is performed by physicians, nurse practitioners, and other trained medical staff.

Compazine (generic name, prochlorperazine): A drug that helps control nausea and vomiting after surgery or chemotherapy.

CT scan: Computed tomography (CT) scans, also called CAT scans, are a radiographic technique that uses a computer to assimilate multiple x-ray images into a two-dimensional cross-sectional image.

Cyst: A nodule that is filled with fluid and is typically benign.

Cytoxan (generic name, cyclophosphamide): A chemotherapy drug commonly used to treat breast cancer and other cancers. Cytoxan first disrupts cancer cells, and then destroys them.

Ductal carcinoma in situ (DCIS): Refers to cases where the cells lining the milk ducts (the channels in the breast that carry milk to the nipple) are cancerous, but stay contained within the ducts without growing through into the surrounding breast tissue. DCIS may be described as precancerous, preinvasive, noninvasive, or intraductal cancer.

Elective: Subject to the choice or decision of the patient or physician. The term is applied to procedures that may be advantageous to the patient but not medically necessary.

ER/PR status: Breast cancer tumors are tested to determine whether they respond to progesterone and estrogen. This is considered ER (estrogen receptor) and PR (progesterone receptor) status, and the result plays a role in the treatment decisions and prognosis. Not all breast cancers are ER/PR positive.

Etiology: The cause and origins of diseases.

HER2 status: The HER2 gene helps control how cells grow, divide, and repair themselves; it is important in the control of abnormal or defective cells that could become cancerous. When breast cancer cells express this gene, it plays a role in the treatment decisions and prognosis. Not all breast cancers are HER2 positive.

Hormones: Chemical substances that have an effect on the activity of a certain organ or organs. Some hormones include progesterone and estrogen.

Immunologist: A physician specialist who treats allergic disease and diseases that involve dysfunction of the immune system.

Infection control measures: When a person is at risk for contracting an infection, such as at times during chemotherapy, measures must be taken to avoid infection. Such measures include avoiding large crowds or public places, avoiding fresh flowers, and not eating raw or uncooked meat or fruits and vegetables that do not have a thick skin.

Invasive ductal carcinoma: A type of breast cancer in which the cancer cells have broken through the milk ducts in the breast.

Lumpectomy: An operation to remove a tumor and an area of margins from a location in the body.

Lymph node: Small bean-shaped organ located along the lymphatic system; lymph nodes are a part of the body's immune system.

Lymph node dissection: Surgical excision of one or more lymph nodes. The purpose of this procedure in cancer surgery is to help predict whether the cancer has spread outside of the original location to another area of the body.

Lymphedema: Swelling of the subcutaneous tissues caused by obstruction of the lymphatic drainage. It results from fluid accumulation and may arise from surgery, radiation, or injury in the area of the lymph nodes or near an area where lymph nodes were removed.

Mammogram: A special imaging examination of the breast using x-rays. The purpose of this test is to detect breast cancer.

Margins: The area of tissue surrounding a tumor when it is removed by surgery. "Clean margins" is a term used to describe tissue that does not contain cancer cells, and indicates that all the cancer has been removed. "Dirty margins" is a term used when the tissue removed contains cancer cells, and is indicative of cancer remaining in the tissue.

Mastectomy: The surgical removal of the breast and surrounding breast tissue.

Menopause: Cessation of menstruation in women, typically occurring naturally around the age of fifty.

Metastases (or metastatic): The spread of cancer from the primary cancer (such as the breast) to other locations in the body (such as the bones, liver, lungs, or brain).

Multifocal: Arising from more than one location. In the case of breast cancer, a tumor or tumors that are in addition to the primary tumor within the breast.

Nadir: When measuring blood counts, this is the point at which the blood counts are at their lowest point.

Neo-adjuvant: Treatment that is given first, with the goal of helping make the next treatment step(s) go more smoothly. For example, chemotherapy, radiation, or hormones may be given before surgery. In breast cancer, this therapy is mainly used to shrink a large tumor so that later on it's easier to excise surgically.

Neonatologist: A physician specialist who cares for infants immediately before birth and during the six-week period after birth.

Occluded: Blocked or closed.

Oncologist: A physician who specializes in the diagnosis, treatment, and rehabilitation of patients with cancer. A "medical oncologist" specializes in the treatment of cancer through the use of chemotherapy agents. A "radiation oncologist" specializes in the treatment of cancer through the use of radiotherapy measures.

Palliative: Measures taken to provide relief, but not meant to cure a condition.

Pathology report: A written report that summarizes the studies performed on tissue removed from the body. The information in the report is useful for determining the best treatment course.

Port-a-Cath: Brand name for a type of small catheter device placed under the skin that empties into a blood vessel and makes it easier to give chemotherapy and to take blood for tests. Also called a "central line."

Premature menopause: Menopause happening at a younger age than usual. This may be caused by an oopherectomy (removal of the ovaries); by the surgical removal of the uterus; or by administering chemicals (medication given to prevent the function of ovaries).

Prophylactic: Preventive measure, such as surgery or medication, to decrease the likelihood of a cancer recurrence or the development of cancer in a location.

Radiation: The use of radiation to kill cancer cells or shrink tumors. Radiation may come from a machine outside the body (external-beam radiation therapy), or it may come from radioactive material placed in the body in the area near cancer cells (internal radiation therapy). Radiation is also often called radiotherapy.

Radiation portal: The area where external radiation enters the body.

Reconstruction: Rebuilding or repairing an area of the body that has been damaged or removed.

Recurrence: When cancer returns after treatment. Cancer may return to the same place as the original cancer site (local recurrence) or in a different part of the body (metastatic recurrence).

Remission: A decrease in or disappearance of signs and symptoms of cancer. In partial remission, some, but not all, signs and symptoms of cancer have disappeared. In complete remission, all signs and symptoms of cancer have disappeared, although cancer cells may still be present in the body.

Tamoxifen (brand name, Nolvadex): An anti-estrogen medication that blocks estrogen from binding to estrogen receptors in the breast. This results in slowing the growth and reproduction of breast cancer cells that are fed by estrogen (ER positive).

Taxol (generic name, paclitaxel): A drug used to treat advanced breast cancer or early breast cancer in patients who have already had chemotherapy. Taxol is classified as a mitotic inhibitor because it interferes with cell division.

Taxotere (generic name, docetaxel): A cancer drug that treats advanced breast cancer in patients who have not responded well to chemotherapy.

Tissue expander: Inflatable reservoirs, usually made of silicone, that are implanted in the area where tissue is needed for surgical reconstruction. In breast cancer, the expanders are typically inserted under the muscle in the chest. After implantation, the reservoir is inflated over several weeks by the injection of saline. Once the tissue has grown, the expander is surgically removed and the expanded skin is used to cover the area being reconstructed.

TRAM flap (transverse rectus abdominis myocutaneous) reconstruction: A type of breast reconstruction whereby the TRAM muscles are used to create a new breast. The TRAM muscles are located in the lower abdomen. In most women there is enough skin, fat, and muscle here to reconstruct a new breast. The tissue can be detached and moved, or the tissue can remain attached as a flap and slid under the skin up to the chest. In both procedures, the abdominal tissue is sewn into place as a new breast. The excess skin and fat that are removed from the lower abdomen are often referred to as a "tummy tuck."

Transesophogeal echo cardiogram (TEE): A special ultrasound test that takes pictures of the heart from a catheter in the esophagus.

Tumor board: A panel of medical experts who make cancer treatment recommendations.

Ultrasound: A type of imaging technique that uses high-frequency sound waves.

Vasculitis: Inflammation of a blood vessel.

Zofran (generic name, ondansetron HCl): A drug that helps relieve nausea and vomiting associated with chemotherapy.

Zoladex (generic name, goserelin acetate): A drug that works by blocking estrogen from the ovaries in women (and blocking testosterone in men), thereby starving these cells.

The glossary definitions were derived from information listed on the following Web sites:

www.breastcancer.org

www.cancerweb.ncl.ac.uk

www.komen.org

www.cancer.org

www.imaginis.com

www.cancergroup.com

Breast Cancer Resources

The American Cancer Society's
Breast Cancer Network
(800) ACS-2345
www.cancer.org
The American Cancer Society is a nationwide community-based voluntary health organization dedicated to eliminating cancer as a major health problem by preventing cancer, saving lives, and diminishing suffering from cancer through research, education, advocacy, and service. The site contains breast cancer basics, information about clinical research trials, and free programs such as the Reach to Recovery program, which provides one-on-one support to newly diagnosed patients.

Breastcancer.org
www.breastcancer.org
Breastcancer.org is a nonprofit organization for breast cancer education. The site contains medical information, research news, a celebrity talking dictionary, pictures of breast cancer, discussion boards, and open chat rooms. The mission of breastcancer.org is to help women and their loved ones make sense of the complex medical and personal information about breast cancer so that they can make the best decisions for their lives.

Fertile Hope
(888) 994-HOPE
www.fertilehope.org

Fertile Hope is a national nonprofit organization dedicated to providing reproductive information, support, and hope to cancer patients whose medical treatments present the risk of infertility.

FORCE
(Facing Our Risk of Cancer Empowered)
www.facingourrisk.org

FORCE is a nonprofit organization for women who are at high risk of developing breast and ovarian cancer because of family history and genetic status and for members of families in which a BRCA gene has been identified (BRCA refers to breast cancer genes).

KidsCope
www.kidscope.org

KidsCope's mission is to help children and families understand the effects of cancer or chemotherapy on a loved one, to provide suggestions for coping, and to develop innovative programs and materials that communicate a message of hope to diverse families coping with this crisis.

Kids Konnected
(800) 899-2866
www.kidskonnected.org

Kids Konnected provides peer support and age-appropriate books for children whose parents have been diagnosed with cancer.

Komen Champions for the Cure™
www.actnowendbreastcancer.org

Komen Champions for the Cure™ is a grassroots program designed to educate Congress, the president, and other policymakers about breast cancer through community involvement.

Lance Armstrong Foundation (LAF)
www.livestrong.org
512-236-8820

The mission of the Lance Armstrong Foundation (LAF) is to inspire and empower people with cancer to live strong. They serve their mission through education, advocacy, public health, and research programs. LAF believes that in the battle with cancer, unity is strength, knowledge is power, and attitude is everything. Founded in 1997 by cancer survivor and champion cyclist Lance Armstrong, the LAF provides the practical information and tools people living with cancer need to live strong.

Living Beyond Breast Cancer (LBBC)
Survivors' Help Line (888-753-LBBC)
www.lbbc.org

The mission of Living Beyond Breast Cancer is to empower all women affected by breast cancer to live as long as possible with the best quality of life. LBBC offers educational information to women affected by breast cancer. Programs include conferences, teleconferences, newsletters, survivors' help line, young survivors' network, and other outreach programs.

Men Against Breast Cancer
www.menagainstbreastcancer.org

Men Against Breast Cancer is the first national nonprofit organization designed to provide targeted support services to educate and empower men to be effective caregivers when breast cancer strikes a female loved one. It also targets and mobilizes men to be active participants in the fight to eradicate breast cancer as a life-threatening disease.

Mothers Supporting Daughters with
Breast Cancer (MSDBC)
www.mothersdaughters.org

This is a national nonprofit organization dedicated to providing support to mothers whose daughters have been diagnosed with breast cancer. This organization offers (at no cost) a mother's handbook and daughter's companion booklet that provides basic information about breast cancer and its treatment as well as some recommended constructive ways for mothers to provide support physically, emotionally, financially, and spiritually. The organization also matches mothers with mother volunteers across the country based on the daughter's (patient's) clinical age at time of diagnosis and anticipated treatment plan.

National Breast Cancer Coalition
www.natlbcc.org

The National Breast Cancer Coalition is a grassroots advocacy effort in the fight against breast cancer. In 1991, the coalition was formed with one mission—to eradicate breast cancer through action and advocacy. To achieve its mission, the National Breast Cancer Coalition focuses on three main goals:

1. *Research:* Increasing appropriations for high-quality, peer-reviewed research and working within the scientific community to focus research on prevention and finding a cure
2. *Access:* Increasing access for all women to high-quality treatment and care, and to breast cancer clinical trials
3. *Influence:* Increasing the influence of women living with breast cancer and other breast cancer activists in the decisionmaking that impacts all issues surrounding breast cancer

National Cancer Institute
www.cancer.gov

The National Cancer Institute (NCI) is a component of the National Institutes of Health (NIH), one of eight agencies that compose the Public Health Service (PHS) in the Department of Health and Human Services (DHHS). The NCI, established under the National Cancer Act of 1937, is the federal government's principal agency for cancer research and training. NCI coordinates the National Cancer Program, which conducts and supports research, training, health information dissemination, and other programs with respect to the cause, diagnosis, prevention, and treatment of cancer, rehabilitation from cancer, and the continuing care of cancer patients and the families of cancer patients. The Web site has up-to-date information on current clinical trials available.

National Coalition for Cancer Survivorship
www.canceradvocacy.org

The National Coalition for Cancer Survivorship is the oldest survivor-led cancer advocacy organization in the country and a highly respected authentic voice at the federal level; the coalition advocates for high-quality cancer care for all Americans and empowers cancer survivors.

National Consortium of Breast Centers
www.breastcare.org

The National Consortium of Breast Center's mission and purpose is to promote excellence in breast health care for the general public through a network of diverse professionals dedicated to the active exchange of ideas and resources. The website also provides a directory of breast centers.

National Patient Advocate Foundation
www.npaf.org

The mission of the National Patient Advocate Foundation is to create avenues of access to insurance funding for evolving therapies, therapeutic agents, and devices for patients through legislative and policy reform.

Patient Advocate Foundation (PAF)
(800) 532-5274
www.patientadvocate.org

Patient Advocate Foundation is a national nonprofit organization that seeks to empower patients to take control of their health care. Case managers work with patients to discover local, state, and federal programs that provide assistance for their individual needs. If you or someone you know needs assistance with their insurer, employer, and/or creditor regarding insurance, job retention, and/or debt crisis matters relative to their diagnosis of life-threatening or debilitating diseases, please contact PAF.

Pregnant with Cancer Network
(800) 743-4471
www.pregnantwithcancer.org
This national network was created by three women who all lived through cancer during pregnancy. The mission of the Pregnant with Cancer Network is to let women who have been diagnosed while pregnant know that they are not alone.

Ribbons of Pink Foundation Fund
www.ribbonsofpink.org
The mission of the Ribbons of Pink Foundation Fund (ROP) is to provide funding for organizations that promote breast health and to support young women who have been diagnosed with breast cancer. Founded in 1999, ROP provides a free e-mail reminder sent on the first day of the month to promote monthly breast self-exams (BSE), and also utilizes a unique tool called the "BSE Tracker" for documenting BSE findings.

Sharsheret
(866) 474-2774
www.sharsheret.org
Sharsheret is a national nonprofit organization of cancer survivors dedicated to addressing the unique challenges facing young Jewish women living with breast cancer. Sharsheret, Hebrew for

"chain," was founded in 2001 by Rochelle Shoretz, who recognized the need for a breast cancer organization that would provide culturally sensitive support for Jewish women after her own diagnosis at the age of twenty-eight.

The Susan G. Komen Breast Cancer Foundation
(800) I'M-AWARE
www.komen.org

For more than twenty years, the Susan G. Komen Breast Cancer Foundation has been a global leader in the fight against breast cancer through its support of innovative research and community-based outreach programs. Working through a network of U.S. and international affiliates and events such as the Komen Race for the Cure®, the Komen Foundation is fighting to eradicate breast cancer as a life-threatening disease by funding research grants and supporting education, screening, and treatment projects in communities around the world.

Susan Love, M.D.
www.susanlovemd.org
Dr. Susan Love's Breast Book: New Edition 2005

This newly updated edition of Dr. Love's book reflects every major new development in breast care, screening, diagnosis, treatment, and research.

Y-ME National Breast Cancer Organization
(800) 221-2141 (twenty-four-hour national hotline)
www.y-me.org

The mission of Y-ME National Breast Cancer Organization is to ensure, through information, empowerment, and peer support, that no one faces breast cancer alone. Services include a twenty-four-hour Y-ME national hotline, a wig and prosthesis bank, advocacy in action, and culturally sensitive breast cancer services and resources.

Young Survival Coalition
  www.youngsurvival.org
  The Young Survival Coalition (YSC) is the only international, nonprofit network of breast cancer survivors and supporters dedicated to the concerns and issues that are unique to young women and breast cancer. Through action, advocacy, and awareness, the YSC seeks to educate the medical, research, breast cancer, and legislative communities and to persuade them to address breast cancer in women forty and under. The YSC also serves as a point of contact for young women living with breast cancer.

About the Authors

Patti Balwanz

Patti Balwanz was working as an information technology (IT) consultant when she found her lump. With a family history of breast cancer, she knew the importance of performing monthly breast self-exams (BSE).

Diagnosed with breast cancer at the age of twenty-four, Patti subsequently had a mastectomy with immediate reconstruction and chemotherapy. Two years after her original diagnosis, Patti was diagnosed with metastatic breast cancer to her bones, lungs, and liver.

During her recurrence, Patti became an advocate for the breast cancer cause, serving as a board officer of the Ribbons of Pink Foundation. Patti openly shared her experience with others, even allowing camera crews to film her while receiving chemotherapy treatments. In August 2001, Patti was honored with the foundation's first "You Are an Inspiration" recognition. Patti attended Southwest Missouri State University (now Missouri State University), where she received a Bachelor of Arts degree in social work and became active in the Alpha Sigma Alpha sorority.

On Saturday, March 29, 2003, at age 29, Patti died at home among friends and family after a four-year battle against breast cancer and a courageous life lived with it.

Jana Peters

Jana Peters was a registered nurse who learned about the importance of performing monthly breast self-exams (BSE) during college, where she attended the University of Kansas and was active in the Delta Delta Delta sorority. She later transferred to Washburn University, from which she graduated with a Bachelor of Science degree in Nursing.

Jana's breast cancer diagnosis came shortly after she became engaged to be married. At twenty-seven years old, while in the midst of planning her wedding, she underwent a mastectomy and chemotherapy. Her cancer spread to her bones eighteen months later, and she has undergone continuous treatments for her cancer progression since that time.

In October 1999, Jana founded the Ribbons of Pink Foundation, a nonprofit organization with the mission of promoting breast health and supporting young breast cancer survivors. She also volunteered for a variety of other breast cancer organizations and events and was selected as one of twenty-five national Yoplait "Champions in the Fight Against Breast Cancer" honorees for 2006.

Jana enjoyed her professional career in the clinical research industry, where she worked for a large biopharmaceutical company in South San Francisco. After a courageous eight-year fight against breast cancer, Jana died on Saturday, December 9, 2006, at age 35.

Jennifer Johnson

Jennifer Johnson is a marketing professional who learned the importance of performing breast self-exams (BSE) while volunteering for the Susan G. Komen Foundation through her college sorority, Zeta Tau Alpha.

Jennifer was diagnosed with breast cancer in 1999 at the age of twenty-seven while five months pregnant with her first child. She subsequently underwent a mastectomy and chemotherapy during the pregnancy. The day following her last chemotherapy treatment, she delivered a healthy baby boy. Proving that life does go on after a breast cancer diagnosis, she and her husband, Matt, welcomed a daughter in April 2003. Jennifer continues to celebrate life cancer-free.

She is active in P.E.O. (a women's philanthropic educational organization) and the United Methodist Church of the Resurrection. She also volunteers for several breast cancer organizations, including the American Cancer Society's Reach to Recovery program, Susan G. Komen for the Cure, the Ribbons of Pink Foundation, the Young Survival Coalition, and the Pregnant with Cancer Network.

Jennifer graduated from Baker University with Bachelor of Science degrees in business marketing and fashion merchandising. Jennifer is a motivational speaker and works for a large telecommunications company in Kansas City. She lives in Overland Park, Kansas, with her husband, Matt, and their two children, Parker and Emma.

Kim Carlos

Kim Carlos is a public affairs and strategic communications consultant who learned about the importance of breast self-exams (BSE) through her good friend and co-author, Patti.

She was diagnosed with breast cancer in 2002 at the age of thirty while in the midst of planning her son's second birthday party. After undergoing eight rounds of chemotherapy, a mastectomy with breast reconstruction, several other surgeries, and treatment for lymphedema, Kim is cancer-free.

Kim is a nationally recognized patient advocate and serves on the Komen National Public Policy Council. She is also past president of the board for the Greater Kansas City Affiliate of the Susan G. Komen for the Cure and helped bring a branch of the Young

Survival Coalition to Kansas City. Kim serves on the Missouri Cancer Consortium Committee, is a member of the American Cancer Society State Advocacy Committee, and is Missouri co-chair for the National Patient Advocate Foundation. She has been honored for her advocacy efforts by *Self* magazine and Lifetime Television and is a member of the National Cancer Survivor Day Speaker's Bureau.

After Kim's breast cancer diagnosis, she decided to focus on her passion full-time and left the practice of law to start her own business, where she focuses on grassroots advocacy, governmental relations, public relations, and motivational speaking. Kim graduated with honors from Missouri State University with a Bachelor of Science degree in marketing and received her Juris Doctorate with honors from the University of Missouri-Kansas City School of Law. She resides in Kansas City, Missouri, with her husband, Scott, and their son, Brandon.

For more information, visit the authors at www.nordiesatnoon.com

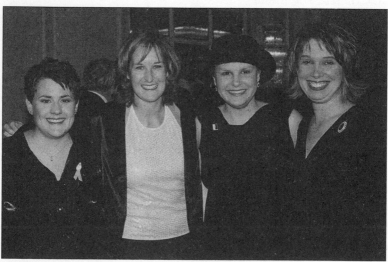

Left to right: Jana Peters, Patti Balwanz, Kim Carlos, Jennifer Johnson

AUTHORS' PHOTOGRAPH BY MYRON CRAMER

Acknowledgments

From the Nordie Girls

Our dream of publishing *Nordie's at Noon* was realized only with the generosity and help of many people. We are grateful to everyone who supported us in achieving this goal. We would like to offer special thanks to those who played a pivotal role.

David Balwanz and Mom and Dad Balwanz: The completion of Patti's writing was possible only because of your efforts. In the process, we adopted David as our brother and we love you like family. Words alone cannot express our gratitude for your dedication and passion for fulfilling the promise we made to Patti—to complete this book. Domisani!

Amie Jew: Thank you for the time you spent writing a thoughtful and insightful foreword. We are also so grateful for the compassionate and exceptional medical care you give to all of your patients—including us.

Marnie Cochran, as our editor of the second edition of our book, we were so excited you shared our vision for the book and invited us to become a part of the Da Capo family. Kate Burke, our publicist extraordinaire. Thanks for all of your great work in helping us spread our message. To the rest of the team at Da Capo Lifelong

Books, you were great to work with and we appreciate your dedication and support. Thank you!

To our amazing estrogen-powered crew who helped the first edition of *Nordie's at Noon* come to fruition: Heidi Potter, Barb Unell, Barbara Bartocci, Pola Firestone, Kirsten McBride, and Vivian Strand. Thank you for guiding us through the publishing process and for polishing our work, and for working within (and meeting) all of our tight timelines.

Lori Jones: Thank you for donating your time and talents to build our website: www.nordiesatnoon.com.

Patti

To Dione Carver and Donna McCool. Dione came up for every chemo session during round one and managed almost monthly visits during round two. Dione, I have no idea what I did to deserve a friend like you, but it was worth whatever it was. Donna, "my ambassador of Kwan," was a constant fixture at my chemo sessions during round two. No day seemed complete unless I shared it with her in some way. A heartfelt thank you to the friends and family who were around when I needed them, shared in my joys and sorrows and helped me find strength I didn't know I had. To my mom and dad, my brother, Grandma, Dr. Jew and Dr. Doane, the Nordie Girls, sorority sisters from near and far, whose light, love, and compassion helped me shine; my extended family, my Bible study group, my many chemo friends and the gracious nurses who made me laugh, my coworkers and supervisors, know that your lives, work, and stories inspired me; Lucy, my number one kid friend; my other friends, too numerous to mention, whose cards, calls, prayers, and kind thoughts helped sustain me and the life in this book, and to my late Grandfather and Grandmother Balwanz and Grandfather Holmes, who taught me how to be tough, love my family, and enjoy the many blessings of life.

Chris: My husband, best friend, and favorite person in the whole world—I am blessed to spend the rest of my life with you. Angi: Thank you for always looking after your little sister and for being the mom to my dear niece, Bronwyn. My Parents: Dad, thank you for being with me, from before, on, and after my diagnosis day, to walking me down the aisle and beyond. Stepmom Patti, thank you for your guidance over the years, and especially for helping me through my difficult cancer treatments—all the while helping me plan the best wedding ever. My Parents In-Law: Ron and Carol, thank you for accepting and loving me as a daughter of your own. My Medical Team (in order of life appearance): Dr. Jew, Dr. Doane, Dr. Coster, Dr. Abdou, Dr. McClung, and Dr. Melisko. The secret is out: you *all* share the title, "The Good Doctor." Final Notables: Nurse Annie, thank you for introducing me to Patti in the infusion room and for being a rebel nurse. Thank you to the rest of my family and friends—you know who you are and I am grateful you are in my life. To all of the ROP board members, volunteers, and sponsors: Your friendships and support have given me more hope and strength than you will ever know. And finally, *thank you,* to my favorite girls (and a guy) to have lunch (and write a book) with: Patti, Jen, Kim, and Dave.

Jen

For my number one support team—my husband, Matt, my parents, Jim and Kaki, and my miracle children, Parker and Emma. Matt, your support was unbelievable. I am blessed to be married to my best friend and soulmate. I look forward to many years to-gether. ILWY. Mom and Dad, thank you for your never-ending support. You have been such wonderful role models of how to be good parents and have a lasting marriage. Parker, you were the reason I fought this with everything I had. Emma, you were such an unexpected and wonderful gift in this journey. I am so blessed to be your mother and I thank God for both of my miracles each day. My extended family, I could always feel your love from miles away. Pam, thank you for the gift of your son and for believing in our project. As an only child, I could never have imagined I would one day have so many sisters through ZTA and P.E.O. Thank you for showing me what sisterhood is all about. I also want to thank my medical team: Dr. Martin, Dr. Custer, and Dr. Hoehn for their amazing efforts. Thank you for making my case seem like your top priority at all times and taking care of me and my precious baby. Dr. Jew, thank you for tender follow-up care and for your efforts with Dr. McClung to make buying swim-suits fun again. To the Nordie Gang, your support and friendship mean the world to me. Who knew what we were getting our-selves into with an idea for a book?

Kim

To my high-school sweetheart, best friend, confidant, and all-time number one supporter, my husband, Scott: I am so blessed to have you in my life. Thank you for always being there for me—I love you more each and every day. Brandon, you are the light of my life and I look forward to the day I dance at your wedding. Mom and Dad—your unconditional love and support has never wavered. Kevin and Kyle—thanks for always being there for your little sis-ter. And the rest of the George family—Debbie, Angie, Brad, Paige, Ben, and Morgan—you all play such a special part in my life. Janice and Leroy, thank you for taking me in as your daughter and for raising an amazing son. My extended family, particularly the Elkin clan, your love and prayers were felt every day. Aunt Barbara, I will continue to fight for a cure in your honor. My Greater Minds friends and the hundreds of other friends who provided me their love and support during this difficult journey—thank you. A special thanks to the wonderful survivors who gave me advice, support, and, most of all, hope. Kristin and Laura—you are the sisters I've always dreamed of having—thank you both for just being you. My entire ASA family—you have shown me that our "sisterhood" is for a lifetime. My Komen and YSC families—thanks for making a difference not only in my life, but in thousands of lives. My medical team—Dr. Jew, Dr. Courtright, Dr. Geier, Dr. Young, Nurse Jenny, Kansas City Cancer Centers, and the amazing staff there—thank you for putting up with my tape recorder and my constant questions—and most of all, thank you for saving my life! And finally, to my Nordie Girls (and little brother, Dave), thank you for letting me be a part of your life—you are each an inspiration to me.